Hippocrates' Maze

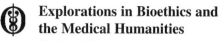 **Explorations in Bioethics and
the Medical Humanities**
Series Editor: James Lindemann Nelson

This series aims to include the most theoretically sophisticated, challenging, and original work being produced in the areas of bioethics, literature and medicine, law and medicine, philosophy of medicine, and history of medicine. *Explorations in Bioethics and the Medical Humanities* also features authoritative contributions to educational contexts and to public discourse on the meaning of health and health care in contemporary culture and on the difficult questions concerning the best directions for biomedicine to take in the future.

Dubious Equalities and Embodied Differences: Cultural Studies on Cosmetic Surgery
by Kathy Davis

Hippocrates' Maze: Ethical Explorations of the Medical Labyrinth
by James Lindemann Nelson

Healing the Self
by Bruce Jennings

Hippocrates' Maze

Ethical Explorations of the Medical Labyrinth

James Lindemann Nelson

ROWMAN & LITTLEFIELD PUBLISHERS, INC.
Lanham • Boulder • New York • Oxford

ROWMAN & LITTLEFIELD PUBLISHERS, INC.

Published in the United States of America
by Rowman & Littlefield Publishers, Inc.
A Member of the Rowman & Littlefield Publishing Group
4720 Boston Way, Lanham, Maryland 20706
www.rowmanlittlefield.com

P.O. Box 317, Oxford OX2 9RU, United Kingdom

ISBN 0-7425-1384-X (alk. paper)—ISBN 0-7425-1385-8 (pbk. : alk. paper)

Printed in the United States of America

♾ ™ The paper used in this publication meets the minimum requirements of
American National Standard for Information Sciences—Permanence of Paper for
Printed Library Materials, ANSI/NISO Z39.48-1992.

For Hilde

Contents

Acknowledgments

While each of the chapters of *Hippocrates' Maze* has its own history and its particular heroes, I take this to be my chance to thank those who have in various ways contributed to the development of the outlook that is expressed throughout the book.

Unlike some of my colleagues who work in what is sometimes referred to as practical or applied ethics, I find much of what's going on in what are often seen as pretty recherché parts of philosophy as fascinating and deeply important. One of the reasons, in fact, why work on topics that emerge from clinical experience so intrigues me is that I think it is simply stuffed with opportunities to contribute to the advancement of research programs in the discipline's core areas. At the same time, part of why very fine-grained exploration of topics in the theory of reference, the metaphysics of personal identity, or the theory of action (for example) strikes me as so worth pursuing is that I think these investigations can make a contribution to our gaining a more adequate sense of the moral situations that confront us in contemporary medicine. I've thought so since the late 1970s, at which time I was writing a dissertation that aimed to mine direct reference theory for implications relevant to ontological disputes in abortion, and, at the same time, to articulate that theory to provide a more plausible account for moral terms such as "person." Dick Hull, now Professor Emeritus of Philosophy at SUNY Buffalo, was enormously encouraging and helpful as I took my first steps along this path, and has been so ever since.

A decade after finishing the dissertation, I found myself at the Hastings Center, a place where one's daily bread is largely earned by convincing funders that discussions about ethical problems are worth paying for. It would be natural to think that the atmosphere would be pretty relentlessly practical in its temper, that it would not be a good place to think about theory—natural, but quite mistaken. Somehow, during my five years there, theoretical inquiry of the kind I wanted to do was always possible, always welcome, always invigorating. I learned an enormous amount from many people who were a part of the Center during my time there; I want to mention here in particular Dan Callahan, Bruce Jennings, Susan Wolf, Philip Boyle, and Erik Parens. Strachan Donnelley's appetite for theory is famous to all who have even the slightest acquaintance with him, and I am grateful to him for all the ways he has supported theoretical work in bioethics.

One of the great boons of working at Hastings is the people that you meet apart from your colleagues, crack thinkers from all over the globe. The person I met at the Center who most influenced my philosophical thinking, however, was a local who does not, alas, count herself a bioethicist at all. Margaret Urban Walker, then of Fordham University, now of Arizona State University, may be surprised to hear this. Nor am I sure how she'll take it. Nonetheless, that's how it seems to me.

Much of this book was first written while I was at the University of Tennessee at Knoxville, where my colleagues and graduate students were as close to being uniformly delightful as can be asserted with any hope of being believed. I am particularly grateful to Allen Dunn, Professor of English and accomplished philosopher, and my former colleague Betsy Postow, a skilled and painstaking philosopher, who helped keep me honest even when I didn't show her my drafts. John Hardwig was a significant influence on my thinking before I ever came to Tennessee, and remains one still.

I have also learned a great deal from my once and present colleagues at Michigan State University, particularly Tom Tomlinson, Len Fleck, and Howard Brody, whose work on "owning, aiming, and sharing" power in bioethics continues to serve as a touchstone for me. I am greatly pleased to think that I have further chances to work with these bioethicists, and with the wonderful assemblage of philosophers, historians, anthropologists, and literary scholars who are doing such fascinating work at the interfaces of their disciplines and health care in East Lansing.

This book was completed during a research year at the Center for the Study of Medical Ethics and Humanities at Duke University, whose director, Jeremy Sugarman—physician, philosopher, and raconteur—expended a great deal of energy and imagination to make our stay possible, fruitful, and great fun. I am very grateful to Duke, and to MSU as well, for jointly supporting the leave.

Eve DeVaro of Rowman & Littlefield was efficient and insightful, to say nothing of showing good judgment, in acquiring this book and in helping me to launch the *Explorations in Bioethics and the Medical Humanities* series in which it appears. I look forward to working with her on *Explorations* for many years.

Hilde Lindemann Nelson read all these chapters in all their many incarnations; if salvation turns out to be the sort of thing that can be earned, that should do it for her. Abstracting from everything else, I am immensely lucky to live with someone doing first-rate philosophical work in areas that both overlap with and interestingly complement my own, who is generous with time and ideas, very encouraging, very tough, and very smart about when to be which, and a highly skilled editor to boot. Of course, what makes me even luckier is that I don't have to abstract from everything else.

The chapters started life as lectures or articles designed for diverse occasions. The opening chapter, "The Meaning of the Act," first took shape around the hallowed conference table at the Hastings Center, during a National Institute for Human Genome Research–funded project on disabilities studies–based critiques of prenatal testing (grant RO1 HG01168–02). As published here, it contains work that first appeared in "Prenatal Diagnosis, Personal Identity and Disability," *Kennedy Institute of Ethics Journal* 10, no. 3 (September 2000): 213–28, and as "The Meaning of the Act: Reflections on the Expressive Meaning of Prenatal Screening," *The Kennedy Institute of Ethics Journal* 8, no. 2 (1998): 165–82.

Early forms of the ideas in the second chapter, "Agency by Proxy," were presented as a plenary lecture at the Twenty-first Annual Meeting of the Austrian Ludwig Wittgenstein Society in Kirchberg, Austria, in August of 1998. The published version of that lecture appeared as "Agency by Proxy," in *Applied Ethics: Proceedings of the 21st International Wittgenstein Symposium*, edited by Peter Kampits and A. Weiberg (Vienna: öbv & hpt, 1999), and material from that version is reprinted by permission.

Chapter 3, "Just Expectations: Family Caregivers, Practical Identities, and Social Justice," originated from an invitation to write on the topic of justice and family caregiving for a collection on justice and health care, and appears here as influenced by my participation in a working group on family caregiving and traumatic brain injury, sponsored by the Hastings Center and the Center for Rehabilitation Ethics of the Chicago Rehabilitation Institute. A somewhat different version of this chapter appeared as "Just Expectations," in *Health Care and Social Justice*, edited by Rosamund Rhodes, Margaret P. Battin, and Anita Silvers (Oxford and New York: Oxford University Press, 2002), reprinted by permission.

An invitation to take part in a working conference on feminist perspectives on women and old age sponsored by the Ethics Center at the University of South Florida prompted the fourth chapter, "Death's Gender," first published in *Mother Time: Women, Aging and Ethics*, edited by Margaret Urban Walker (Lanham, Md.: Rowman & Littlefield, 1999).

Chapter 5, "Everything Includes Itself in Power," started out as a plenary lecture for a conference in Youngstown, Ohio, in 1995, marking the appearance of the second edition of Tristram Englehardt's *Foundations of Bioethics*. An earlier published version appeared as "'Everything Includes Itself in Power': Power and Coherence in Engelhardt's *Foundations of Bioethics*," in *Reading Engelhardt*, edited by Brendan Minogue, Gabriel Palmer-Fernández, and James Regan (Dordrecht, The Netherlands: Kluwer Academic Publishers, 1997). Material from that version is here reprinted by permission.

Chapter 6, "A Duty to Donate? Selves, Societies, and Organ Procurement," arose from an invitation to contribute a chapter to a volume on the ethics of organ transplantation. In its present form, it is influenced by a lecture I was invited to give at Albany Medical College in 2000, a talk I delivered at a meeting of the Feminist Approaches to Bioethics meeting in London in the same year, and a very pleasant lunch I shared in at the Center for Ethics and Humanities in the Life Sciences as Michigan State University in 2001. The earlier version was published as "A Duty to Donate? Selves, Societies and Organ Procurement," in *The Ethics of Organ Donation and Transplantation*, edited by Wayne Shelton and John Balint (Greenwich, Conn.: Elseveier Press, 2001), reprinted by permission.

The final chapter, "Cloning, Families, and the Reproduction of Persons," results from a submission to the National Bioethics Advisory Commission during its deliberations on cloning in 1997. The version delivered to NBAC was published as "Cloning, Families and the Reproduction of Persons," in the *Valparaiso Law Review* 32, no. 2 (1998): 715–25, reprinted by permission.

J.L.N.
East Lansing, Michigan
October 2002

Introduction

So Daedalus made the innumerable paths of deception (*innumeras errore vias*), and he was barely able to return to the entrance: so deceptive was the house (*tanta est fallacia tecti*).[1]

Ovid

Like the maze Daedalus made to contain the Minotaur, the intricacies of contemporary health care also confuse those who might be thought of as its makers, or at least as its native inhabitants—physicians, nurses, therapists, and allied health care providers, administrators, insurers, and health policy analysts. You can imagine—or perhaps recall—the utter bewilderment often experienced by those caught up in health care as patients or family members. The sheer number of the decisions faced, the Byzantine bureaucratic tangles in putting them into practice, the importance of what hinges on these choices, and the awareness that many options will lead down paths of deception with monsters waiting at their ends is daunting, to say no more.

From the start, medicine has been a curious business. It seeks out sick and vulnerable people and convinces them to make themselves even more vulnerable, both physically and emotionally, to someone who may well be a complete stranger. It persuades these sick people to follow that stranger's advice, the point of which is often poorly understood, and to do things that make them feel still worse or are downright dangerous. For these services, handsome payment is expected. Perhaps as a result—perhaps as an effort to create an impersonal, institutional reservoir of trust—medicine has a venerable tradition of attention to ethics as an integral part of good quality care.

But in our time, medicine's dazzling technological power and its formidable social heft have forced the realization that its traditional moral moorings no longer go deeply enough. It's not demeaning to doctors to observe that it is no longer responsible to rely solely on the good character of health care providers and the wisdom of medicine's indigenous moral traditions to guide what health care is now and what it will become. Hippocrates' Oath isn't enough to guide us through Hippocrates' maze. It is widely acknowledged that good practice requires not only explicit attention to ethics, but a richer and more powerful set of normative and interpretive resources than it can supply on its own.

And this, of course, is just what bioethics has sought to provide over the last three or four decades of the twentieth century. Drawing on philosophy, theology, law, literature, and history, as well as the social scientific disciplines, scholars have developed, debated, and refined strategies for practical reasoning tailored to clinical contexts. They have also put together many thoughtfully motivated positions on moral issues emerging in almost every aspect of health care.

Bioethics understood in this way is often subsumed under the broader rubric of "applied" ethics. (One now hears occasionally of "applied humanities" as well.) Applied ethics, as I understand the idea, is a fairly commodious notion. It is not limited, for example, to what is sometimes characterized and often criticized as "deductivism" in bioethics methodology—the notion that one can resolve moral quandaries by deducing prescriptions for appropriate behavior from moral principles and statements describing the relevant facts. Applied ethics is, however, a well-enough defined notion to convey a pretty clear division of moral labor. Philosophers and other scholars deal with abstract ethical problems, structuring moral theories to handle them; the goal is primarily to improve the quality of the theories. Bioethicists and other applied ethicists interpret the implications of these theories for real-world, real-time problems, sometimes tailoring the theories to make them more user-friendly to practitioners and always (at least ideally) paying careful attention to the nuances of the context and the subtleties of the practice.

This book aims to exemplify an alternative approach. In this volume, I examine a fairly diverse sample of bioethics' staple problems: prenatal genetic diagnosis, proxy decision making, justice in the allocation of resources demanded by health needs, death, the theoretical foundations of the field, organ procurement, and reproductive cloning. I address some of the considerable and vigorously expanding literature on these problems and offer my own contributions to practical resolutions as well. But the unifying architectonic for the book is not a matter of subjects treated or even of conclusions reached. The coordinating motif is, rather, a metabioethical matter—an effort to reason via examples to the conclusion that the applied ethics model is inadequate for reliably orienting ourselves within the maze, and that, further, the model hides the opportunities that the maze offers for a deeper understanding of human conditions. If the inability of "indigenous" medical ethics to illuminate bioethical issues has been widely recognized for over two decades, it is now time to recognize that "applied" bioethics won't do the job either.

In some important respects, there is nothing particularly new about this notion. For about as long as bioethics has been a discernible practice, there have been people uncomfortable with the idea that practical moral problems in medicine (or elsewhere) could be solved by pulling theories out of moral philosophy, letting them grind away at the facts, and extracting a conclusion thence. What I maintain—explicitly here and implicitly throughout the book—is that this discomfort has sources and dimensions that need further articulation. What's more, we need to see that bioethicists who don't think they extract answers from theory in any lock-step way are still overly influenced by the applied model. What I intend these chapters to exemplify, then, are three related but distinguishable reasons why the model neither does full justice to what bioethics is and what it might become, nor to the problems and opportunities it confronts.

The first reason is that good bioethics, even in its clinical uses, needs more and better theory, not limited, simplified versions of a small portion of what philosophy and other "home disciplines" are developing. By "theory," I don't necessarily mean highly structured edifices of covering laws waiting for initial conditions to be plugged in, and I certainly don't mean to call for any kind of strictly deductive application of theory to some practical domain. This is not a plea that bioethics should become more resolutely Millian, Kantian, or Rawlsian. Rather, my use of "theory" refers to something on the order of disciplined, rigorous, and sophisticated bodies of thought. My point here is that many bioethicists have been too quick to limit the range of their theoretical gleaning to ethical theory, and too ready to assume that practicality and pluralism imply that only the broad outlines of moral theory are going to be of much use. I hope to demonstrate the utility of bolder forms of bioethical *bricolage*, of employing cutting-edge philosophical work in different clinical and policy contexts.

The chapter on prenatal genetic diagnosis, "The Meaning of the Act," is perhaps the book's most sustained effort to make this idea attractive. There I assess the objection that prenatal testing, followed by abortion, sends disparaging messages about the worth of people currently living with the conditions the tests seek to detect. I think this "expressivist objection" is a very important concern, well worth careful considerations, and yet not in the end convincing. To understand why the objection is not persuasive, general reflection on what is involved in sending a message, informed by contemporary philosophy of language, is in order. Further, while the objection quite sensibly tries to distinguish between benign ways of forestalling disabilities— e.g., prevention or treatment—and the ways it regards as insulting, this too fails. To see why, we must sort out questions in the metaphysics of personal identity.

Similar kinds of strategies are employed in "Agency by Proxy," the chapter in which I discuss making health care decisions for those unable to make them on their own. The orthodoxy on this matter has it that explicitly authorized or otherwise appropriately situated people can report treatment preferences that incapacitated patients entertained earlier, or, in the absence of clearly applicable preferences, proxies can draw on their acquaintance with the patient's values and desires to make decisions. I augment recent philosophical work on the theory of agency with a view known as "active externalism" to argue that some people—chiefly drawn from among those sometimes called "bonded intimates"—can not only report a patient's preferences or convey her values, but can creatively and flexibly make decisions on the patient's behalf, drawing on a shared deliberative viewpoint, not merely on supposed special knowledge of specific preferences or general values.

In "Just Expectations: Family Caregivers, Practical Identities, and Social Justice in the Provision of Health Care," I turn to recent moral theoretic work on the connection between a person's conception of herself and her moral duties and opportunities. I argue on that basis that the increasing burdens the health care system slides onto the backs of care-giving family members gives them a claim on social resources that is roughly as weighty as claims advanced on the behalf of the ill.

Results from areas of philosophy other than moral theory, or from bioethically underexplored parts of moral theory, are employed elsewhere in the book. But if this were the book's only departure from more standard practices, I might reasonably be seen not so much as offering an alternative to the idea that the fundamental methodological principle in bioethics is the application of theory, but rather as urging us not to be skimpy about what we try to harvest. The concern that my interest is really in more and better application, rather than in doing something aimed further from the orthodox model, sets the stage for my second reason for being unhappy about seeing bioethics as simply and solely an applied activity. Health care contexts are not merely places where bioethicists may distribute the distillates of theory learned elsewhere. Rather, the clinic is a good place to do philosophy and is brimming with challenges useful to the development of theory.

This claim questions an idea that seems to be at the heart of the applied model: the whole point of bioethics, when one gets right down to it, is to figure out how to give good advice to doctors and perhaps to patients, families, policy makers, and other practitioners as well. But bioethics can be more than a guide to the practically perplexed. It can also make significant contributions to the traditional agendas of philosophy and other humanities disciplines as well, aiding in the development of those basic ideas with which we understand ourselves and direct our actions.

In the chapter, "Death's Gender," for instance, the aim is to contribute to a very old and persistently troubling question—is death a harm to us? Epicurus and Lucretius argued that death does not harm us at all ("What is death to us? When we are, death is not; when death is, we are not"). Thomas Nagel argues that it harms everyone in a dire and categorical way ("a bad end is in store for us all"). Some bioethicists have responded to the endemic shortages in medical resources that might extend a patient's life by developing what is in effect a third position: the idea that, while death is a harm, its harmfulness varies with the age of the decedent. I take off from that idea, arguing that the harm of death may be sensitive to other human characteristics as well—gender, in particular. The practical implications of that insight are not thoroughly worked out in the present chapter—that's a horse for another race—though I try to sketch out some features of our social responses to mortality that may be unfortunate for their neglect of how death is "gendered." But in general, I am confident that drawing upon the challenges of understanding and negotiating complex social practices to develop better philosophical accounts of death, or the nature of the self, or of action, or of justice, will rebound back to the practices and offer us more insightful, better defensible notions of how to act within them. At the same time, the idea, if correct, is valuable in itself, as a contribution to our understanding of our mortality, surely one of the fundamental conditions of human life.

I strongly suspect that this benign feedback loop, deepening understanding and refining action as we move from practice to theory to practice, will hold for disciplines other than philosophy. Scholars in medicine and literature, for instance, have explored how various narratives can play a role in the education of physicians and medical students, how they can speak to the affect, enlarge imagination, and hone perception more powerfully than can discursive argumentation. They have also argued that forms of reasoning in health care are typically more narrative than, say, hypothetical or deductive, more like making sense of a story than like solving an equation. But there remains, I think, the task of asking what seeing clinical practice as a richly imagined, densely written text can tell us about the character, methods, and aims of literary studies. What might it add to debates about whether interpretation is still an appropriate task of literary scholars, for example? How might involvement in the clinic provide ways of reading texts that deal with medical situations—and nonmedical situations too, perhaps—that are not readily available from the study or the library.

I try to show here, then, that an understanding of bioethics that conceptualizes it solely as an applied matter, a source of insight that theorists provide for practitioners, misses an important interactive dimension: the insight available to theorists from close engagement with practitioners. The third reason that the applied model is too simple builds on this theme of interactivity, expanding it beyond theory to more comprehensive matters: contemporary medicine contributes importantly to the ongoing restructuring in how people think of themselves as individuals, as members of communities, and as beings of a certain kind.

This thought involves rejecting a wholly instrumental understanding of health care's role in social life. Contemporary medicine and its attendant disciplines are simply too complex and powerful a part of our culture to plausibly construe them as merely features of life that respond to what we want and who we are, quite apart from their contributions to how our identities, values, and preferences are assembled. Medicine creates, sculpts, or distorts the wants it tries to satisfy; it contributes to the shaping of selves.[2]

Something allied to this idea has become commonplace in contemporary culture. It's often said, and sometimes even carefully argued, that our new understanding of the genome, along with, perhaps, new psychopharmaceuticals or other neuroscientific findings and interventions, threaten to change our very natures, ushering us into what has been called a "posthuman future."[3] For example, consider some of the basic ideas appealed to in various accounts of moral reasoning. If we think, say, of the promotion of welfare as a fundamental goal of the ethical life, medicine and its attendant sciences may not merely have a role in its promotion (or frustration), but in changing our notion of what welfare is or includes. If scrupulous respect for autonomy is the hallmark of morality, what happens as medicine and the life sciences alter our view of ourselves as free and responsible moral agents? And if a shared and distinctive human nature is a normative touchstone, how should we respond to the possibility that medical interventions may change that nature, and change it in ways to which only some human beings have access?

In each of these cases, the concern is that the basic normative metric—e.g., welfare, autonomy, human nature—may be significantly altered by medicine. To the extent that such alteration goes on, we're left in a poor position to assess the changes, as our moral measuring sticks themselves become rubbery. One response, of course, is to try to slam on the brakes, but given the nature of the problem, it's hard to see what plausible, principled motivation that strategy might have, to say nothing about its dim prospects for success.

But it isn't these scenarios that most pique my interest. Part of my aim in this book is to argue that there is nothing so conspicuous about genetic medicine, psychopharmacology, or neuroscience; medicine as such is a major player among the many social practices that have been reshaping the identities offered to us, and hence our nature as social beings, for quite some time now. In the chapter, " 'Everything Includes Itself in Power,' " I try to show that the tough questions medicine poses puts pressure on the idea that ethical reasoning is something we may be able to engage in profitably together that by deepening the divides in our pluralistic culture on issues of great practical and moral significance, difficult bioethical questions make distressingly stark the limits of rational discourse to provide a generally acceptable way of responding to those problems.

But another part of my aim is to deflect the thought that medically mediated changes in individuals, or even in general natures, are uniformly something we ought to avoid resolutely, or to lament when unavoidable. In "A Duty to Donate? Selves, Societies, and Organ Procurement," I ponder what happens when simple arguments collide with complex feelings, and examine neglected analogies between gestation and organ provision, exploring the interplay between the conception we entertain of our boundaries and the ability of medical advances to destabilize those boundaries. I argue that there are good reasons to welcome that destabilization, and even to celebrate the ways in which organ sharing makes possible a new form of human intimacy. And in "Cloning, Families, and the Reproduction of Persons," I explore both how interest in reproductive cloning—like interest in other forms of technologically assisted reproduction—has tended to neglect the extent to which bringing new people into the world is a fundamentally social task, while at the same time pointing to ways in which cloning might promote currently subordinated forms of familial diversity that are ethically desirable.

In sum, then, the book works not so much to offer the field a brand new way to make sense of itself, as to shift to the foreground a theme in the self-understanding of bioethics that has been somewhat obscured by its concerns with demonstrating its practical importance, striving for a defensible place in medical education's curricular battles and a seat around those tables that determine how policy and practice in this enormously important dimension of everyday life will go on. These struggles continue, but bioethics has achieved for itself a far from negligible degree of institutional stability. It's well positioned now to speak to our reflective, as well as our regulatory, needs and to help us gain the kind of clear overview we need to negotiate so cunning a maze.

NOTES

1. The Labyrinth, a web-based resource maintained by Georgetown University's Medieval Studies Program, directed me to *Metamorphoses* 8.166–68, Ovid's characterization of the maze, which I use as my epigram. See labyrinth.georgetown.edu (accessed May 10, 2002).

2. Even a comparatively minor social force like bioethics itself needs to keep an eye on its social impact. It wouldn't hurt a bit if we were more reflectively aware of how bioethics' own characteristic activities and results both articulate rationally defensible goals and constraints and impress people into a regimen of values that they may not recognize as fully their own. A very thoughtful argument for this kind of distortion is Carl Schneider's *The Practice of Autonomy* (Oxford: Oxford University Press, 1998). Hilde Lindemann Nelson and I explore the same point in a way less finely focused on autonomy in *The Patient in the Family* (New York: Routledge, 1995).

3. The phrase is owing to Frances Fukuyama, *Our Posthuman Future: Consequences of the Biotechnology Revolution* (New York: Farrar, Straus and Giroux, 2002). For a more sophisticated discussion of the possibility that the ability to manipulate the human genome may undermine structural features of contemporary theoretical options in our understanding of justice, see Allen Buchanan, Dan W. Brock, Norman Daniels, and Daniel Wickler, *From Chance to Choice: Genetics & Justice* (Cambridge and New York: Cambridge University Press, 2000).

1

The Meaning of the Act
Relationship, Meaning, and Identity in Prenatal Genetic Screening

Is it correct for someone to say: 'When I gave you this rule, I meant you to . . . in this case'? Even if he did not think of this case at all as he gave the rule? Of course it is correct. For 'to mean it' did not mean: to think of it. But now the problem is: how are we to judge whether someone meant such-and-such?

Wittgenstein

If you visit your state capital and make your way to the seat of government, you'll typically find two flags flying, emblems of both nation and state. But until the summer of 2000, residents of South Carolina had a bonus. Three flags fluttered colorfully over the dome of the State House in Columbus: the Stars and Stripes; the palm and crescent moon of the state flag; and the banner of the Confederate States of America, the Stars and Bars.

The presence or absence of a piece of colored cloth on a pole might seem irrelevant to the central concerns of state government: it doesn't affect the Medicaid budget, teacher salaries, or road repair. But whether or not that third flag flew in Columbus inspired heated demonstrations, numerous petitions, both action and pointed inaction in the State Senate and House of Representatives, boycotts, and a good deal of bitterness. For some South Carolinians, the official display of the Confederate flag duly honored a rich heritage for which their ancestors fought and died. For others, it sent the despicable message that killing and dying in the defense of slavery is a heritage worth honoring.

The kind of dispute illustrated by flying the Stars and Bars over the

State House is not rare. Human actions express meanings as readily as they have causal consequences, and people often care deeply about what those meanings are. Another site where the meaning of particular acts has become hotly contested is in the medical genetics clinic, where prenatal testing for genetic conditions that may give rise to disabilities has itself become something of a red flag. Several disability theorists and activists claim that the use of medical technologies to detect flaws in parental genes or fetuses, leading to the avoidance of conception or abortion, is just a way of saying "we don't want your kind here"—a technologized medium for a type of hate speech. The philosopher and disabilities theorist Susan Wendell makes the point in virtually these terms when she says, "The widespread use of selective abortion to reduce the number of people born with disabilities . . . sends a message to children and adults with disabilities, especially people who have genetic or prenatal disabilities, that 'we do not want any more like you.'"[1] Laura Hershey puts a similar point just as bluntly: "I believe the choice to abort a disabled fetus represents a rejection of children who have disabilities."[2] In the words of Marsha Saxton, "The message at the heart of widespread selective abortion on the basis of prenatal diagnosis is the greatest insult: some of us are 'too flawed' in our very DNA to exist; we are unworthy of being born."[3]

Are Hershey, Wendell, Saxton, and others of like mind correct in construing efforts to avoid the birth of such children as an insult to people with disabilities? This question merits attention. According people the respect they are due is a matter of general moral importance, and we ought be especially scrupulous when people who have endured a history of negligence and abuse claim that they are yet again being demeaned. Attending to this complaint will also alert us to something about the character of bioethical questions not widely enough realized. The emergence of bioethical issues is generally tied to new technologies coming on line, and it might be thought that the "prenatal testing/selective abortion" issue is just another instance of the general trend. But, as I hope to show here, what makes genetic screening problematic is to an important degree a result of shifts in how we understand who we are, what most fundamentally contributes to our identities, how we make our identities plain to others, and what affects their uptake of the messages we send. Without such shifts, the complaint pressed by Hershey, Saxton, Wendell, and other disabilities scholars and activists does not arise. Without better understanding the complexities of human identity and human expression, we will not be able to understand, or to answer it responsibly.

DOING AND MEANING

Performing amniocentesis is a different sort of deed from hoisting a banner; abortions are not flags. The semantic force of diagnostic tests and pregnancy termination is not well defined within our shared symbol systems, and whether there are clear messages to be found in such practices needs more careful consideration than it typically gets. A characteristically authoritative paper by Allen Buchanan, "Choosing Who Will Be Disabled: Genetic Intervention and the Morality of Inclusion," is a good place to start, largely because it assesses this complaint by means of an explicit account of what has to be the case for an action to express a meaning.[4]

Buchanan calls the view that genetic testing and abortion send negative messages the "expressivist objection." He puts it like so:

[T]he commitment to developing modes of intervention to correct, ameliorate or prevent genetic defects expresses (and presupposes) negative, extremely damaging judgments about the value of disabled persons.[5]

Buchanan draws this version of the objection from the work of the "radical disabilities rights position," particularly as developed in an issues paper by the International League of Societies for Persons with Mental Handicaps.[6] The objection leaves him unimpressed, and in this formulation, that's hardly surprising. As it stands, it suggests that developing even the simplest intervention to cure or prevent even the most horrendous disease is morally dubious, and surely that comes close to a reductio ad absurdum. But the expressivist objection takes on much more force if it is restricted to interventions which, rather than preventing, curing, or ameliorating an individual's disease, prevent or eliminate a diseased individual. As Adrienne Asch and Gail Gellner put it, "What differentiates preventing disability by abortion from preventing it by immunization is that the abortion indicates that the disability makes the child unacceptable."[7]

Later I want to return to the idea that abortion and immunization (or other therapies) are readily distinguishable as means to prevent disability; I am not persuaded that this trick can be pulled off—and hence, the reductio avoided—as easily as Asch and Gellner think. For the present, however, I assume that proponents of the argument are not committed to regarding therapies (or preventive strategies, like seat belt and helmet laws) as sending insulting messages to disabled people; the problem for the moment is abortion.

Buchanan raises what is clearly a key question: just how does an abortion "indicate" that disabled children—and by implication, disabled people—are unacceptable? As he sees it, the claim that an action conveys a meaning only has force if the actors involved meet two conditions. The first concerns the *content* of their beliefs. In order for an action to convey a certain meaning, the actor must have the beliefs purportedly expressed by the action. Thus, a person deciding to avoid the birth of a baby with disabilities must believe something disparaging about people with disabilities—for example, that life with the disabilities in question would not be worth living, or that only "perfect individuals" (i.e., those without disabilities) are worthy of being born. The second condition is that those beliefs must play a certain *role* in a person's decision making. In the case of a person who avoids having children she expects might have disabilities, her decision must either be motivated by such beliefs, or cannot be a rational decision absent her accepting such convictions.

But, as Buchanan points out, choosing to abort or to avoid procreation as a result of prenatal or preconception testing does not imply having passed this two-part test. To argue convincingly that these actions convey such a negative meaning, it would have to be shown that people making these decisions have beliefs that demean the disabled, and are motivated by those beliefs. But this flatly is not the case; many motivations can be imagined for trying to avoid the birth of a baby with disabilities, and many reasons can be provided for such action that do not involve such beliefs as "a life with disabilities is not worth living," or "only the 'perfect' should be born." One may, for example, "simply wish to be spared avoidable and serious strains on one's marriage or on one's family" or "one may wish to avoid putting additional pressure on limited social resources to support disabled individuals."[8]

Buchanan thinks that people are perfectly at liberty to avoid having children on such grounds, since doing so wouldn't violate anyone's rights; there is, after all, "no existing individual who has rights that might be violated."[9] Avoiding conception clearly doesn't violate anyone's rights, and abortion violates rights only if fetuses have a right to be born, a view Buchanan thinks highly implausible. Yet even were it the case that fetuses had such a right, the expressivist objection to abortion would be beside the point. On this assumption, abortions as such would be (at least prima facie) wrong because fetuses are rights holders, not because (some) abortions would express disrespectful messages about the disabled.[10]

I think that Buchanan's strategy of examining the conditions required for behavior to convey a sense is key to assessing the expressivist objection. I also must agree that, at the end of the day, the expressivist objection does not succeed in showing that avoiding the conception or birth of children with disabilities necessarily expresses messages that disparage people with disabilities. However, I think the expressivist objection is more complex than Buchanan allows. In what follows, I will try to show why the objection has more to it than Buchanan thinks, why it ultimately fails as a grounds for justifying restricting access to testing and abortion, and what it has to teach nonetheless.

THE SEMANTICS OF STERILIZATION

Shortly after the birth of my third child—this would be in 1982—I decided to get sterilized. In retrospect, I think I made a good decision, all things considered. At the time, though, there was one thing that did worry me a bit. It wasn't the thought that I might change my mind about wanting more children. Even if I had a change of heart, I would likely still believe that considerations of global and intergenerational justice (to say nothing of justice within the family) entailed that I was not entitled to bring more children into the world. My worry was a different one. It was what deliberately destroying my ability to procreate would say about my attitude to Eric, Laura, and Melissa, the three children I already had.

What I wanted, of course, was to live so as to convey plainly and consistently to my kids that they were deeply loved and most welcome. But I wondered whether that message would be distorted or deflected by the steps I had taken to make as sure as I possibly could that I would never have another child. Even more disturbingly, I wondered whether my desire to be sterilized was really fully consistent with the welcoming attitude I professed.

As it happened, I don't think any of my children have ever had a moment's anxiety or discomfort about my vasectomy. What's more, I ended up parenting six children, which only goes to show how fate can get a good chuckle out of our attempts to control the dimensions of our lives. But although my concerns turned out to be, so far as I can tell, misplaced, I don't believe that they were hopelessly confused.

I tell this story because I think it illustrates how people can intelligibly have concerns related to the expressive character of their reproductive decisions that do not fall within Buchanan's construal of this matter, and are not stilled by his arguments. In being concerned about the expressive character of my sterilization, I was concerned about what my motivations and reasons *really* were—I didn't assume that they were necessarily altogether manifest to me. Simply checking the aspects of my beliefs and motives that were readily accessible to my awareness didn't settle the matter. Nor was I troubled about the moral claims of the children I might have had had I not been sterilized; that's not a confusion to which I was tempted. The discordant, disrespectful message I feared I might be sending was not directed to merely possible individuals; I was concerned that it might be addressed to, and perhaps received by, quite real individuals—my children.

So if we might call Buchanan's criticism of the expressivist objection, the "many meanings" rejoinder, we might call the moral of my story, the "meanings aren't (necessarily) manifest" rebuttal. Yet perhaps rather than regard my story as a counterexample to his analysis, we might say that his analysis captures a dimension of what it is for a piece of behavior to express a sense. In one of his contributions to the multiply authored *From Chance to Choice: Genetics and Justice*, he seems to allow for just this possibility, imagining a proponent of the expressivist argument making this claim:

> Even if the decision to use genetic interventions to prevent disabilities does not *necessarily* express negative attitudes, such attitudes are all too common in society [and] are part of the motivation for the willingness of develop and use genetic interventions. We should not encourage these attitudes by using social resources to create vehicles for their expression and perpetuation. (Italics added)[11]

This is just the possibility I want to put squarely on the table: that neither the in-principle existence of many possible, benign motivations for testing and aborting, nor the lack of consciously held objectionable beliefs, shows that disrespectful messages are not being conveyed by the practice of prenatal testing and termination.

ABORTION, EXPRESSIVITY, AND ASCH'S "ANY / PARTICULAR" DISTINCTION

So a successful challenge to the expressivist objection must do more than judge it against Buchanan's strict content/role conditions, and more, too, than dismiss the concern altogether on the ground that fetuses are merely possible people who possess no rights. But the objection is not out of the woods yet. Even if it passes semantic muster (still a large "if") those who press it are going to have to be clearer about what it actually implies for practice, and why. Should access to the diagnostic technologies that provide women with information about their fetuses be restricted? Should there be *no* such testing, or testing only for conditions incompatible with life, such as Tay-Sachs? Or should women seeking to use such tests, or to act on the basis of what the tests reveal, be compelled to learn more about what's involved in caring for children with disabilities, before they are allowed to end their pregnancies?[12] These questions underscore that supporters of the expressivist objection have more work to do in clarifying the moral weight of the offense to people with disabilities, and how it stacks up against competing values.

But there is another hurdle that has to be cleared first: showing that abortions that have an objectionable expressive character can be distinguished from those that do not. This is a tricky business. Many friends of the expressivist argument are not foes of abortion *tout court* and want to resist other efforts to impede women's control over their own reproductive lives. Can the expressivist objection cleanly sort out the dubious prenatal-diagnosis-inspired abortions from all the rest, which are to be regarded as "just" the woman's business?

Adrienne Asch has made an important effort to defend such a distinction. She notes that some women who find themselves pregnant wish to end the pregnancy for reasons that do not seem to involve properties of the fetus they are carrying; such women would end any pregnancy, no matter what properties the fetus possessed, because of considerations that pertain to their own situations. They are merely rejecting pregnancy or parenthood as such. As fetuses are not rights holders, and as no woman should be forced to remain pregnant against her will, abortions in such instances are morally unproblematic.

Other women wish to end a pregnancy on the basis of the properties they believe to be possessed by the particular fetus they are carrying. Such people have made something of a commitment to parenthood; they would be willing to parent some children in some contexts. But now they are picking and choosing among possible recipients of their parental care, on the basis of what those fetuses would be like were they to come into the world. A woman who was prepared to become a mother to the child that would have developed from this fetus now changes her mind on the basis of merely a single piece of information, a single trait possessed by the fetus—that it would be a person with disabilities. Again, such picking and choosing may not violate any right held by the fetus, but it does express a negative attitude toward those who are already morally considerable, and are like the fetus in the relevant respect.[13]

While I think this is a very interesting effort to distinguish between "properly private" abortions and those that raise wider moral questions, I haven't been able to bring myself to think it does the work it seems to be trying to do. In part, my reservation is rooted in my story: if any reproductive decision is a matter of rejecting *any* possible child, as opposed to some particular child or child-precursor, sterilization would seem to be it. And yet, I was concerned about what my decision *represented*, about what I was saying about the worth of a child. Why could not, therefore, abortions aimed at any child be seen as disparaging to all of us?

Perhaps an adequate account of what must be the case for nonlinguistic behavior to convey sense would show that my concern here was confused. But such an account has not been forthcoming from Asch or anyone else who has employed the expressivist objection. Nor has Buchanan's reconstruction, resting on beliefs or motivations apparent to the agent, resolved the matter either, at least if it is possible for a person to be moved by considerations not all of which may be perfectly clear to her. Remaining at an intuitive level, then, it seems as though even very general kinds of reproductive decisions, such as sterilization, or the abortion of "any" fetus, might well have at least some of the same kind of implications for wider constituencies that more particular acts do. That is, they might express morally objectionable attitudes. Restricting the force of the expressivist objection to disabilities seems ad hoc.

There is a possible response here. Sterilization—at least, if we exclude the case of sterilization motivated by concerns about one's chances of procreating a child with disabilities—may have many meanings, some objectionable, some not. The same might be said about the abortion of "just any" fetus. One might so despise disabilities that the bare chance that a child might be born with handicaps would be enough to motivate an abortion, but this would be an odd circumstance, to say no more. It is morally responsible to give the benefit of the doubt to people seeking sterilization, or the abortion of any fetus they might be carrying, as there is so much their action might mean. But if a woman were to end a previously wanted pregnancy on finding out that she is carrying a fetus who she can anticipate will become a child with disabilities, there is, so this rejoinder might proceed, only one way to take that.

Buchanan has anticipated this response. He points out that a woman choosing an abortion after prenatal testing need not be saying to herself, "people with disabilities have no right to exist." Rather, she need only believe that fetuses with presumed genetic defects have no right to be born (a circumstance they share with all other fetuses), and she might well be motivated by concern about the effect that raising a child with special needs might have on other features of her life, or on other people with disabilities, for that matter. But again, a riposte is possible. Such concerns themselves bespeak an objectionable attitude. If the woman believed her pregnancy would issue in a "normal" child, the stresses involved in rearing would have been acceptable. Not so with the stresses involved in caring for a disabled child. What can be concluded except that the person whose decision pivots on this consideration is saying that people with disabilities aren't worth the time and trouble that they require?

The short answer is that many things could be concluded. The woman may believe that the character of the stresses involved in nurturing a child with disabilities would be markedly different, in degree or in kind, from those she was willing to undertake. Further, if choosing not to parent a child with disabilities entailed a belief that people with disabilities aren't worth the support they may require simply to live, then the vast majority of people who are capable of being parents, and yet have not sought to adopt disabled children, must be committed to such a repugnant belief as well, and this, too, looks uncomfortably like a reductio.

But this last point, at least, won't seem a satisfying reply to the objectors; the pregnant woman who refuses to bear and subsequently nurture a child she believes will have disabilities is pointedly and vividly refusing an opportunity with which she is directly presented, and that surely appears to make a difference. So, rather than continue to discuss whether women in such a position might not have adequate reasons for ending pregnancies that do not demean people with disabilities, I want, for sake of argument, to leave open the possibility that abortions subsequent to prenatal testing might express objectionable messages to disabled people and return to the question of whether or not abortions otherwise motivated might also send equally objectionable messages. I focus on whether abortions done for reasons other than specific genetic indications are really so "nonparticular" as Asch requires.

Women who choose not to complete a pregnancy will, at least in very many instances, have reasons for making this decision. For example, a woman may decide that her family is quite large enough. This seems precisely the sort of thing that Asch would likely regard as a matter of "the situation of the woman," rather than of the "characteristics of the fetus or would-be child." The difficulty, however, is that if this woman should become pregnant, the fetus she is carrying does seem to have a property—a single trait—that is squarely involved in her decision to abort: the property of being the "n + 1" fetus, where "n" was this woman's highest acceptable number. Suppose her "n" is three; does that suggest that this woman is sending a message that she devalues fourth-borns, or that she is expressing contempt, or some other morally objectionable attitude, about large families? While it is not easy to imagine how we could keep women from knowing how many children they have (the technology for making such determinations—counting—is already in wide use) the options for proponents of large families are not exhausted. They might insist that that this woman study accounts of the joys of mothering more than three children, or visit happy homes with big families before she is allowed to obtain her abortion.

Imagine now a woman who decides not to complete her pregnancy because she thinks herself too poor to have a child. The fetus she aborts, then, seems to stand to the property "indigence" much as a fetus with a genetic defect stands to the property "disability." That property, then, becomes her reason for the abortion. Does this action say something disturbing about this woman's attitude regarding poverty and poor children? Should poor women undergo special education about raising poor children before they abort? Are the stresses of raising such children enough in excess of those involved in raising middle-class children to justify the abortion without the need to assume that the woman does not sufficiently value poor people?

We can also readily imagine instances in which a woman is initially ambivalent about her pregnancy, or even welcomes the idea of becoming a mother, but changes her mind during pregnancy. She loses her job, or her partner, or her health. In such cases one could raise the same kinds of questions about what her reproductive decision says about poor kids, or kids raised by single mothers, or by ill mothers, with the added circumstance that such a person was clearly not saying she didn't want to be a parent at all; she just didn't want to be a parent when it turned out that the child she would be bearing would have a certain trait.

Are these cases really on all fours with disability cases? Here's a tempting reason to think they are different: a sharp line can be drawn between "the situation of the woman" and the "characteristics of the fetus" because genetically based disabilities are what philosophers call "monadic" properties, ones that inhere in the fetus itself, depending on no consideration of context. Further, such properties may be seen as essential to the fetus's basic identity as the thing that it is. Being a fourth-born, or being poor, in distinction, are relational properties, features that characterize a child only in a given context, and that hold only contingently of the individuals in question. Someone might say that disabilities are "intrinsic" properties, whereas properties like birth order or economic status are not intrinsic.

In fact, someone has. In dissenting from my account of the "fourth-born" case, Nancy Press has written:

> Although one's place in the family birth order may come to leave a mark on a child, it is not an intrinsic attribute of that child, but rather of that pregnancy. Put up for adoption and raised in another family, the fourth-born biological child may become the first-born adopted child. But a disability is intrinsic to the child. A fetus definitively diagnosed with a disability will have the disability, whatever family raises it.[14]

But drawing this distinction turns out not to be helpful to proponents of the view that testing and aborting carry a morally objectionable message. To start, Press leaves unexplained why this intrinsic/nonintrinsic distinction is supposed to vindicate the expressivist argument. On its face, it does not seem relevant. True, a person is fourth-born only via her relationship to others, as a person is poor only via her place in a particular economic system. The relational character of a property does not, however, prevent it from being the basis of disparaging attitudes aimed at the person who possesses it; just consider the way indigent people are treated in the contemporary U.S. The expressivist argument takes what plausibility it has not from the supposed intrinsic character of disability, but from the social reception of disabled people; that reception has been disgraceful, but it is not disabled people alone who have suffered disgraceful treatment. So even if we allow that disabilities are intrinsic properties, while birth-order and economic status are relational properties, nothing seems to follow. People have been enormously creative in finding reasons for insulting others. A little thing like the metaphysical distinction between intrinsic and relational properties is hardly going to stop them.

What strikes me as most curious about Press's claim, however, is not its apparent irrelevance to the argument, but the fact that it runs directly counter to one of the most important lessons that the disabilities movement has to teach—namely, that disabilities are, in very important measure, relational. While perhaps "having three copies of one's twenty-first chromosome" counts as an intrinsic property, "having Down's Syndrome" does not—at least, if "intrinsic" means that a property makes whatever impact it does independently of its social context. As Asch has put it:

> If some portion of the difficulty of disability stems from the biological limitations, the majority does not and is in fact socially structured. . . . [E]ven those characteristics we label as "disabling" are at least partly socially determined . . . [and] . . . disability's all-too-frequent consequences of isolation, deprivation, powerlessness, dependence, and low social status are far from inevitable and within society's power to change.[15]

I conclude then that the "any/particular" distinction fails as a basis upon which to separate abortions that may remain private from those which have social implications because of what they seem to say, and that, as a consequence, it will be difficult to maintain a position that objects only to abortions motivated by the prospect of disability, and let the others pass. But even still, the expressivist argument, or at least the concerns that give rise to it, is not wholly stilled. For the possibility remains that, as a matter of fact, people who abort pregnancies on grounds of concerns about disabilities too often harbor offensive attitudes toward disabled people, or are negligently ignorant about them, and that such attitudes are part of the explanation of their reproductive decisions. And it is open as well that termination decisions for other reasons—poverty, or partnerlessness, say—less often involve objectionable attitudes. I also want to explore the possibility that the meaning of an act may not be tied so tightly to what is going on in the head of the actor as Buchanan's account suggests—an action may convey a meaning whether or not the actor is aware of the beliefs that motive her actions. Finally, I will return to the matter of whether treatment could be excused from sending a negative message, if testing does.

INTENTION AND MEANING

I believe the discussion up to this point has undermined the view that a person's decision to employ preconceptual or prenatal testing, and to abort on the basis of those findings, can *only* be taken as expressions of disrespect for people with disabilities. Buchanan has pointed out other possible motives, and I, in the spirit of a reductio, have tried to show that one could make an equally good case for saying that virtually any abortion expresses disrespect for people who share with the fetus the traits that motivated the woman to end the pregnancy. But neither Buchanan nor I have precluded the possibility that some or many acts of testing and abortion, if not *necessarily* expressing objectionable meanings, *may* do so. The question is whether or not in fact they do. To address this question, I want to go back again to my own case and try to get clearer about what I was worrying about back in 1982.

I was concerned that my children might take what I did to be an indication that I didn't want them in my life as wholeheartedly as I do. I was afraid that they might mistake my intentions. Now, as it turned out, this was not a realistic fear. It might have made sense for my children to interpret my behavior in this way if I had been otherwise abusive or neglectful. If I had tried to make their lives harder than they needed to be, or showed in a myriad of ways that I just didn't want to be bothered with them, then sterilization might well have been seen as yet another kind of repudiation. This is, of course, a halting analogy to the relationship between people with disabilities and the general society. It does hint why advocates for people with disabilities might be very concerned about what prenatal diagnosis and abortion mean to the women who seek out such services, as well as to the society that sponsors their availability. But it also suggests that the proper response to this concern may have little directly to do with reproductive decision making and a great deal to do with how people with disabilities are incorporated into social life.

But there are other possibilities, too. I was worried then about what my actions expressed to myself. Did they reveal that, in a way I was hiding even from myself, I really harbored negative feelings about my children, about the ways they had complicated my life, added to my burdens, reduced my disposable income? Here, of course, the crucial problem wouldn't be what my children took from my actions, but rather what was there to be taken. This is more complicated, because it suggests that what my actions mean is not altogether a matter of what I want or consciously intend them to mean. My actions may express things about me—perhaps hateful things—even if nobody picks them up, things that even I cannot be sure about. Analogously, women facing decisions to continue or abort pregnancies may think of themselves as perfectly accepting of people with disabilities, when in fact they may have feelings and beliefs of which they are not fully aware, and would not reflectively endorse if they were fully aware of them, and which at the same time affect their decisions to terminate.

There is no reason to dismiss this possibility out of hand. But again, what seems to follow is that the problem isn't testing or screening programs, or abortions for genetic indications, but rather generally entertained beliefs, attitudes, and policies toward people with disabilities in general. After all, not getting a vasectomy—still less, being prevented from getting a vasectomy—would not in itself have made me a better parent. In trying to right beliefs, attitudes, and policies disparaging of people with disabilities, interfering with reproductive liberties—an activity about whose expressive force we may also have reason to wonder—may be just the wrong thing to do. If the goal is to reduce the chance that people often harbor false and disrespectful beliefs about people with disabilities, it isn't clear why educational efforts ought to concentrate on a practice in which, relative to the whole population, few people will engage, trying to force them to reconsider a kind of behavior that is likely going to be of the first importance to their lives, yet, insofar as it affects people with disabilities, has only an expressive impact.

On this account, the complex of prenatal diagnosis and abortion is at worst the symptom, not the disease. It would seem more reasonable to educate more widely, focusing particularly on areas in which ignorance and disrespect will play themselves out directly in the lives of people with disabilities. What we need is not pregnant women being compelled to attend to certain information as they consider whether or not to go on with their pregnancies, but people generally being presented with more information—including more novels, movies, and television programs—featuring people with disabilities realistically. We need more books such as Michael Bérubé's powerful *Life As We Know It*, that make the rich and complex reality of life as a parent of a child with a disability more vivid to more people.[16]

SOCIAL MEANINGS

My conclusions thus far: individual actions of obtaining various tests and making various reproductive decisions proceed from many motives and with many different understandings; any meanings such actions express will be fraught with ambiguity. Testing and termination decisions are not necessarily disparaging of the disabled, and insofar as the motives or beliefs that prompt them are disrespectful of people with disabilities, the most effective way to challenge them is probably not by making access to abortion harder, or by scheduling mandatory counseling sessions.

But rather than the individual choices of pregnant women, consider the general social practice of developing and disseminating more and more tests for more and more conditions: Does that practice not express a clearer and plainly objectionable meaning, one that needs to be dealt with directly by trying to stop or at least dramatically restructure prenatal and preconceptual testing?

A glance back to Columbia, South Carolina, might be useful here. After an enormous struggle, the Stars and Bars continue to wave—not over the State House, though, but rather over a memorial to confederate soldiers on the State House grounds. In seeking to have the flag removed from atop the State House, was Governor Jim Hodges committed to the view that the individuals who advocated flying the flag were motivated by racist beliefs, or that their actions were only intelligible in the light of such beliefs? Possibly, but not likely, particularly given his willingness to allow the flag to fly on state property after all. Perhaps his action was just an attempt to defuse a controversy by coming up with a politically viable compromise, one not committed to any particular view of what that flag expresses, much less any view of what has to be the case for a flag to express anything whatsoever.

But there is, I think, another possibility. The issue between those who are offended by the display of the flag of a slave society, and those who wish to continue flying it as a symbol of a rich heritage, is not exhausted by considerations of sincerity or even transparency about what those who wish it to fly mean in so doing. The flying of the Confederate flag *over the seat of state government* might convey an offensive meaning, even if no one involved in running it up the pole did so under the influence of offensive thoughts, whether manifest to them or latent in their subconsciousnesses.

Some recent currents in the philosophy of language suggest that meaning and intention are indeed more complexly related. For example, in a footnote in the *Philosophical Investigations*, Wittgenstein writes: "Can I say 'bububu' and mean 'If it doesn't rain I shall go for a walk'?"[17] While it is brash to be sure about what any of Wittgenstein's remarks mean, I think he clearly expects his imagined interlocutor to say, "No, I can't," and to learn something about meaning from this thought experiment. I take Wittgenstein here to be drawing our attention to the extent to which meaning is a social phenomenon, not determined solely by what goes on, as we might say, in our heads. Of course, even if Wittgenstein is right, all he shows is that meaning isn't completely determined by our own intentions; for all he's said here, it might be necessary to my meaningfully using the phrase, "If it doesn't rain I shall go for a walk," that I have certain accompanying beliefs and intentions. Still, Wittgenstein's work, and others in like vein, does at least hint that practices might have expressive content in a way that is not solely a function of our beliefs.

What does determine meaning then? One possible response, again associated with Wittgenstein, is that the meaning of a symbol is in many cases a matter of how it is used, its role in a publicly shareable system of symbols. It is on the basis of considerations of this sort that flying the Stars and Bars over a state house could be reasonably taken to constitute an expression of contempt for African Americans, even if there were no conscious or unconscious racist beliefs or feelings motivating its (contemporary) appearance. The meaning of that symbol, it might be maintained, stems both from the conventional role of flags as symbols for collectivities and their aspirations, and from this particular type of flag's place in America's tragic history of slavery and the defense of slavery. It cannot, then, be used as a state symbol (as opposed, say, to a museum exhibit) without expressing contempt for African Americans, any more than we can say "bububu" and mean "If it doesn't rain I shall go for a walk."

So, the possibility that abortion as a response to disability expresses contempt for the disabled seems opened anew, since it now seems at least possible that "selective abortions," or policies that promote their occurrence, can have semantic properties in a way that does not essentially refer to mental states, open or hidden, of those choosing to terminate pregnancies or institute the relevant prenatal testing practices. Such practices take place against a very disturbing historical backdrop concerning the place to which people with disabilities have been assigned in American society. Given this, the widespread, partly publicly funded development and employment of prenatal and preconceptual tests, and pregnancy terminations because of their results, might seem to be the equivalent of flying the Confederate Battle Flag over the South Carolina State House.

I, however, remain of the view that even considered as a social practice, the meaning of testing and abortion remain both vague and ambiguous, and insofar as this practice does enfold objectionable meanings, the way to unseat them is not by restricting individual access to information and medical services, nor even to curtail the development of prenatal or preconceptual tests for disabilities. Reproductive policies and practices motivated by disability considerations occupy a different semantic position than do the Stars and Bars.

Consider what Wittgenstein has to say immediately after the "bububu" passage. "It is only in a language that I can mean something by something."[18] Again, this is not a perfectly clear claim, particularly because it isn't evident just what would be countenanced as a language and what would not. But this sentence does call attention to how languages are settled social practices that, among other things, include devices for selecting sounds, images, or movements that more or less precisely have semantic significance, and that (interacting with context) thereby keep ambiguity and vagueness under some control. And it is the absence of these elements in individual acts or general practices of screening and abortion for disability that lead me to doubt whether such behavior expresses morally objectionable attitudes independent of the attitudes of individuals who engage in them.

Flags, and where and how they are flown, are unambiguously symbols; it doesn't stretch matters too far to say that they have a role in a language. While there is surely room for dispute about just what might be symbolized by a particular instance of display, any such dispute takes place against the backdrop of an entrenched practice of seeing flags as expressive of a nation and of what characterizes that nation most fundamentally. One simply couldn't say that flying the Battle Flag over the state house means whatever "we" want it to mean; if the South Carolina legislature had passed a proclamation saying, "the flying of Stars and Bars over the State House Dome has nothing whatsoever to do with slavery or racism," that would hardly have settled the question of what it means to fly that flag in that place.

Programs of screening and abortion, on the other hand, do not take place against a settled practice of seeing them as expressing what a community is and with what it identifies. It is not, unfortunately, inconceivable that certain kinds of social backdrops—say, states with Nazi-style policies—might make it unmistakable just what such programs aim at. But this sort of situation would be analogous to the person who seeks an abortion out of a general and professed policy of expressing contempt for children at every possible turn. As things stand, thankfully, there is no reason to see screening programs as emblematic of a Nazi-like state, whose policies are shot through with virulent contempt for people with disabilities. There are other, more plausible ways of understanding both the social deployment and the individual use of preconceptual and prenatal testing.

CHARACTERIZATION, REIDENTIFICATION, AND CONSTRUCTION

Thus far, I have presented the expressivist argument as presupposing certain views about the nature of meaning, and I have used considerations from the philosophy of language to try to rebut it. But at base the argument does not reflect an interest among disabilities scholars and activists in semantics; its deepest ground, in my view, is a view about disability as an identity, an identity that creates a sense of kinship between currently disabled people and "the next generation" of the disabled. The expressivist objection to abortion as a response to beliefs about possible disabilities befalling a fetus emerges from this notion of affinity. I will wind up my consideration of the argument then, by considering disability as an identity.

Earlier, I tried to show that it is going to be hard to restrict this objection solely to disabilities; if abortions motivated by the results of prenatal tests indeed send unambiguously disparaging messages to people with disabilities, abortions otherwise prompted will have their expressive victims as well. Here, I want to argue that it will be hard to restrict the objection solely to abortion. I will argue that if expressivistic considerations pertain to abortion, they must also pertain to efforts to avoid the conception of a fetus facing such probabilities, or to therapeutic responses that might eliminate the conditions that may result in the disability.

A defender of the expressivist argument against this apparent implication would have to show that destroying a fetus to prevent the existence of someone with a disability is morally worse, all things being equal, than preventing the occurrence of disabling traits that someone would otherwise have had. The point of departure for this defense will be the claim already quoted from Asch and Geller: "[W]hat differentiates preventing disability by abortion from preventing it by immunization is that the abortion indicates that the disability makes the child unacceptable"[19]—presumably because the abortion eliminates the child (or child-precursor) while the immunization does not.

To reiterate, Asch and Geller do not base this argument on a conviction that aborting fetuses is morally problematic as such, but rather on their view that the elimination of a fetus who would face disability if born expresses a message that disparages disabled people, while eliminating the disability the child would face does not. But it seems to me that this position in fact requires the view that the termination of fetal life is morally problematic as such. Without attributing some particular disvalue to abortion, it is hard to understand the difference on expressivist grounds between eliminating the dysfunction and eliminating the dysfunctional individual. If abortion on the basis of prenatal diagnosis sends a "we don't want your kind here" message, why would therapeutic interventions not do so as well—and the more successful the therapies are, the more effective the message? If abortion to avoid parenting a child with disabling conditions involves making a decision based on a single trait, would not efforts to cure or prevent disability also involve value assessments based on a single trait? If testing and abortion militate against social acceptance of disabilities as examples of human variation, why would testing and treatment not do so as well?

The claim that abortion and therapy may be expressively equivalent is a key challenge to the "pro-choice" proponent of the expressivist argument. It also makes trouble for Nancy Press's view that critics of the argument mistake who it is who sends the disparaging message.[20] The sender, as Press sees it, is not the individual woman making her individual decision; it is instead the society that mobilizes its resources to provide prenatal testing, confidently assumed to lead to abortion in the majority of cases in which testing detects anomalies. I have already claimed that this conclusion is implausible: considered either as an individual choice, or as a social policy, genetic testing is not sufficiently well-regulated semantically to send a tolerably unambiguous message to anyone. But this social version of the expressivist argument becomes yet more implausible if it cannot be distinguished from the claim that mobilizing social resources to support research and therapy aimed at eliminating the impact of disabling traits also disparages disabled people.

I now want to argue that at least some imaginable in utero interventions, aimed at prevention or therapy, might actually change the numerical identity of the fetus, so that it is no longer the same individual who would have been born without those interventions. In other words, the potentially disabled individual is eliminated by (some) therapeutic interventions just as she or he would have been by abortion. This result implies that Asch and Geller's distinction between responding to fetal anomalies via abortion and responding to such anomalies via prevention or therapy does not do the work they hoped it would.

PREVENTION

That avoiding or repairing fetal anomalies may actually change the identity of the fetus (and/or the person it may become) might seem a startling claim, but it is supported by at least three lines of thought. Call the first line of thought "the prevention argument." The prevention argument rests on the idea, often associated with Saul Kripke's work[21] but anticipated by the eighteenth-century novelist Laurence Sterne in *Tristram Shandy*,[22] that the identity of a particular person is necessarily a function of the joining of precisely those gametes that did in fact join in that particular person's case, along with the observation that even extremely small changes in the course of events can alter which sperm unites with the ovum in question.

Now consider Barbara, a woman interested in having a child. We can imagine Barbara adopting different courses of action in the light of her interest. She might be unimpressed by what she sees as the hype surrounding pregnancy and, hence, gives no thought to her folic acid intake, or any special exercise program, or eating in any particular way.

But we can also imagine Barbara acting differently. In this alternative possible world, she is very careful to be sure that she eats according to a prescribed regimen, takes the recommended supplements, and so forth. It is quite possible that these differences in her routine from world to world will slightly change the incidence, the timing, or even the position of intercourse with her partner, with the result that different sperm inseminate the same ova, with the further result that different children are born to her depending on whether or not she takes the kinds of precautions against disability just described.

Taking those precautions does not merely mean that she has improved the chances that her child will escape, say, a neural tube problem; taking the precautions means that she very likely may have a different child than she otherwise would have had. Prevention, then, can preclude the existence of the child-who-would-have-been-disabled, and not just of the disability-the-child-would-have-had, just as effectively as does abortion.

It might be rejoined that whether disparaging messages are sent is not a matter of arcane metaphysics, but of what people actually believe they are doing. Generally when women (at least women who aren't philosophers) take folic acid and so forth, either they are aiming directly at fostering the health of the child they will have, or, at most, the content of their belief cannot be easily parsed between "taking care that their child be healthy" and "taking care that they have a healthy child." This ambiguity derails the disparaging message. In contrast, when women follow testing with abortions, matters are much plainer. Whatever their motivations, they know they are terminating their pregnancies due, at least in part, to the high probability that the fetuses would face disabilities were they to become children.

One difficulty with this rejoinder is that it hinges on the assumption that metaphysical ignorance is invincible—that no one ever reads *Tristram Shandy*, or Saul Kripke, or takes to heart what she learns in Introduction to Philosophy. Would advocates of the expressivist argument have to oppose preconceptual prevention strategies for those who happen to believe that such strategies may result in an entirely different child than the one who otherwise would have been born?

But the rejoinder has a more important problem. Suppose it were brought to the attention of women considering becoming pregnant that various preconception activities designed to reduce the chances of disabilities might actually change which child they ended up conceiving, not merely how healthy that child was likely to be. Providing this information would dispel the ambiguity about the implication of preventive measures that the defenders of the prevention/abortion distinction claim will deflect the disparaging message. Someone still inclined to use, say, a folic acid supplement, would have to allow that she was willing to take steps to prevent bringing into the world a child who might otherwise have been born with spina bifida, and not just willing to help a given child avoid this condition.

Setting this scenario allows a crucial question to be asked: Is it likely that most women, on getting this information and considering these alternatives, would decide to forgo using the supplements? If not, then the attitudes and actions of women using preventive measures should be as objectionable to these critics as the attitudes and actions of those using abortion, because those women would be just as willing to avoid the birth of a disabled child as to reduce the chance that their child will have disabilities. They would be, in effect, indifferent between the two possibilities.

In my view, this indifference would not be morally problematic, but it is hard to see how proponents of the expressivist argument could share this position. If those convinced by the argument see the actual use of prevention as innocent, they must think that women using preventive strategies are not indifferent about these possible implications of their choice, but rather just confused about the whole matter, and if women really knew what they might be doing in taking folic acid, they would stop taking it. This strikes me as implausible.

THERAPY

Now to the second line of thought—call it "the therapy argument." The therapy argument imagines that genetic therapies are available for in utero treatment of fetuses with diagnosable genetic anomalies. Here, the concern is that altering the genetic structure of a fetus, at least if done early enough, may itself be enough to change the numerical identity of the being. This is allied to the intuition supporting the prevention argument. If one does generally accept that each of us must necessarily be the result of precisely those gametes that we did in fact result from, then that belief may rest, at least in part, on the view that the causal sequences that begin at conception are so basic that any alteration in them will ramify repeatedly through development, inducing so many changes that beings who do not share the same gametes cannot be identical across possible worlds—that is to say, a state of affairs in which some other of my father's sperm had fertilized my mother's ovum than the one that actually did, is not a state of affairs into which I would have been born. If a genetic therapy applied early in fetal development were to generate a similarly cascading train of differences, then therapy is in no better position than prevention to identify the person born subsequent to the treatment with the person who otherwise would have been born.

It might be responded that the most the therapy argument shows is that some, but not all, imaginable interventions threaten identity. If a pregnant woman were to agree to have a shunt installed in her fetus to relieve hydrocephaly, for example, her action would seem to raise none of these metaphysical issues. I think this must be granted. It does not seem plausible in such cases to imagine that the numerical identity of the object in question—the living human fetus, later baby—has altered. However, if the condition repaired would have been serious and pervasive enough, it might well have structured so much of the person's life that, in the absence of those conditions, there is an important sense in which the resulting person would not be the same. And this leads us to a third line of thought, which harkens back to my earlier discussion of disability as a relational property: call it "the social construction argument."

SOCIAL CONSTRUCTION

This line of thought draws on the notion that in addition to questions about what makes a being the same over time—the "reidentification question"—the personal identity issue also contains questions about what makes me the person I in fact am—the "characterization question," to use terms of art supplied by Marya Schechtman in her *Constitution of Selves*.[23] Answers to the characterization question are given by noting features of the narratives in which a person is embedded, narratives that must surely involve in significant ways how different people are configured by the societies in which they find themselves.[24]

If human identities are, in this sense, socially constructed, then, from the perspective of the characterization question, numerically the same individual could be different persons in different social worlds. If a person were ensconced in sufficiently different social narratives, due to her having or failing to have a sufficiently severe disabling condition, she might well be a different person as socially constructed with a disabled identity from the person she would be if she were socially constructed as someone whose abilities were considered normal. Even if it were false that, for example, removing the extra genetic material at chromosome twenty-one resulted in a change in numerical identity of the fetus in question, losing a future as a child with Down's Syndrome seems a very plausible candidate for a change in personal identity in Schechtman's sense.

To help solidify these ideas, consider the following hypothetical: suppose that parents can select the sex of their children via hormonal interventions early in pregnancy. At least if one supposes that the process affects only phenotypic characteristics, a fetus would survive the procedure with its numerical identity intact. One might say of a couple contemplating such an intervention that they are contrasting a possible future in which their fetus is born a girl, and grows to be a woman, with another future, in which one and the same fetus is born a boy, and grows to be a man. Despite the bodily continuity that secures numerical identity here, there seems a different sense of personal identity according to which one would want to say—at least in a society in which gender determines as much about a person as it does in ours—that the person subjected to the intervention is so different from what she or he otherwise would have been as not to be the same person at all.

This example exploits the point that gender, despite its close relation to conceptions of personal identity in the lives of many people, is in significant measure socially constructed—as are disabilities. It is possible to imagine the significance of gender otherwise. In some possible worlds, a difference in shape of genitalia, or endocrinological differences, or differences in reproductive roles, might have no implications for one's sense of identity—these things might be human variations with no more significance than hair or eye color. But in this world, we order things differently.

In some possible worlds, similarly, differences in physical traits other than gender might have little or no salience with respect to personal identity—the significance of an inability to hear is likely going to be much different for a deaf child born into present-day middle America than for a deaf child born into a world like the nineteenth-century Martha's Vineyard described in Nora Ellen Groce's *Everyone Here Spoke Sign Language*.[25] As things stand, however, at least some disabilities—perhaps most plausibly those that are pervasive, visible, and involve cognitive or affective impairment—can structure so much of the way a person experiences the world, and so much about how the world experiences the person, that the presence or absence of those conditions may well be relevant to matters of personal identity, in the characterization sense. Again, the proponent of the expressivist objection seems uncomfortably placed to distinguish between preventing or treating a disability and aborting a potentially disabled fetus following prenatal testing.

CONCLUSIONS: CONTEXT, CONTEXT, CONTEXT

What, as a matter of fact, does stand behind the social and professional interest in prenatal screening, testing, and abortion? The failure to take people with disabilities with full moral seriousness? Or an effort to increase the effective reproductive choices of women and try to give them a further measure of control over how they will live their lives? How do such practices fare in the competition for social support vis-à-vis efforts to construct a society more welcoming to people with disabilities or more empowering of women? Are they leading to the kind of situation feared by Bérubé, where, rather than allowing people more control over the circumstances in which they take up the challenges of parenting, prenatal testing and abortion are seen as part of what it means to be a good parent and a responsible citizen?[26] Screening and aborting do not wear their meaning on their sleeves. If we want to work out how to come to grips with their popularity in our world, then questions like these are the right ones to ask. Tracking them down will likely lead to mixed answers, leaving us doubtful whether such practices express anything clearly enough to be seen as having a meaning. The meanings of decisions, practices, and policies that involve screening and abortion cannot be determined outside the context of a broader set of decisions, practices, and policies as they affect people with disabilities, as well as women and family life more generally. Examining that context will no doubt reveal some disturbing things. But in the end, the attempt to improve social attitudes and practices regarding people with disabilities by putting pressure on prenatal screening and pregnancy termination ought not be construed as a matter of principle on the model of a right to be untroubled by hate speech, or by a racist symbol displayed over the seat of government. It may be, rather, that we need to ask the strategic question of where to invest energies to increase the probability of admirable changes in the way we live our lives. Looked at in this way, tactics other than intervening in women's reproductive decision making seem both less problematic and more meaningful.[27]

ACKNOWLEDGMENTS

Research for this essay was supported by grant ROIHG01168–02, "Prenatal Testing for Genetic Disabilities," made by the ELSI division of the National Human Genome Research Institute to the Hastings Center for a research project exploring the various "disabilities studies" perspectives on prenatal testing. I am grateful to Erik Parens, principal investigator, and to all members of the Hastings Center project, from whom I have learned a great deal (although by no means enough, as many will think). I am also grateful to participants at a meeting of the Society for Disabilities Studies held on May 22, 1997, in Minneapolis, for their very valuable comments on a very early draft of this chapter. Versions of this material were also given as talks at the second annual meeting of the American Society for Bioethics and Humanities, Philadelphia, Pa.; the summer bioethics conference sponsored by the Center for Bioethics at the University of Otago, Dunedin, New Zealand; and the Department of Philosophy at Michigan State

University. I appreciate the invitations to present my work at these venues and the insights of my interlocutors. Several of the participants in my NEH Summer Seminar, "Bioethics in Particular," held during the summer of 2000, also participated in a discussion about these issues, and I thank them for the thoughts they shared with me, and thank as well the Endowment for bringing scholars together for opportunities of this kind. Hilde Lindemann Nelson, the codirector of the seminar, has for many years been both generous and challenging in helping me think through what means what. I'm also grateful to Cynthia B. Cohen and Elizabeth Leibold McCloskey for their close attention to later drafts of version of this material originally published in *The Kennedy Institute of Ethics Journal*, and to Carol Mason Spicer, *KIEJ* editor, for her willingness to let me continue to think through these problems in the pages of her journal.

NOTES

1. Susan Wendell, *The Rejected Body* (New York: Routledge, 1996), 153.
2. Laura Hershey, "Choosing Disabilities," *Ms. Magazine* (July/August 1994): 30.
3. Marsha Saxton, "Disability Rights and Selective Abortion," in *Abortion Wars: A Half Century of Struggle, 1950–2000*, ed. Rickie Solinger (Berkeley and Los Angeles: University of California Press, 1998), 37–95.
4. Allen Buchanan, "Choosing Who Will Be Disabled: Genetic Intervention and the Morality of Inclusion," *Social Philosophy and Policy* 13 (1996): 18–46.
5. Buchanan, "Choosing Who Will Be Disabled," 28.
6. L'Institute Roeher, *Just Technology?* (North York, Ontario: L'Institute Roeher, 1994).
7. Adrienne Asch and Gail Gellner, "Feminism, Bioethics and Genetics," in *Feminism and Bioethics: Beyond Reproduction*, ed. Susan M. Wolf (Oxford and New York: Oxford University Press, 1996), 318–50.
8. Buchanan, "Choosing Who Will Be Disabled," 31.
9. Buchanan, "Choosing Who Will Be Disabled," 31.
10. Buchanan, "Choosing Who Will Be Disabled," 35.
11. Allen Buchanan, Dan W. Brock, Norman Daniels, and Daniel Wickler, *From Chance to Choice: Genetics & Justice* (Cambridge: Cambridge University Press, 2000), 279.
12. Adrienne Asch makes a suggestion of this sort in her "Reproductive Technology and Disability," in *Reproductive Laws for the 1990's*, ed. Sherill Cohen and Nadine Taub (Clifton, N.J.: Humana Press, 1988), 69–124.
13. Asch, "Reproductive Technology and Disability," 82. It should be

underscored that Asch has been clear that, while richer information about the rewards as well as burdens of rearing children with disabilities should be provided women contemplating abortion after prenatal diagnosis, "a woman has the right to decide about her body and her life and to terminate a pregnancy for this or any other reason." *Women With Disabilities: Essays in Psychology, Culture and Politics*, ed. Michelle Fine and Adrienne Asch (Philadelphia, Pa.: Temple University Press, 1988), 302.

14. Nancy Press, "Assessing the Expressive Character of Prenatal Testing: The Choices Made or the Choices Made Available?" in *Prenatal Testing and Disability Rights*, ed. Erik Parens and Adrienne Asch (Washington, D.C.: Georgetown University Press, 2001), 215.

15. Asch, "Reproductive Technology and Disability," 82. Curiously, Asch seems to forget this germinal point in a more recent essay, in which she endorses Press's claim that " 'fourth-borness' does not inhere in the fetus/ child in the same way that disability does; the fourth-born child could just as easily have been the first or only child if adopted into another family." (Asch, "Why I Haven't Changed My Mind about Prenatal Diagnosis: Reflections and Refinements," in Parens and Asch, *Prenatal Testing*, 237.) But contrast a child born with a hearing impairment to hearing parents with that same child adopted by deaf parents who are deeply involved in Deaf culture. At the very least, some people—including many of those most deeply reflective about disabilities—will want to claim that the child in the second scenario is not disabled.

16. Michael Bérubé, *Life as We Know It: A Father, a Family and an Exceptional Child* (New York: Pantheon, 1996).

17. Ludwig Wittgenstein, *Philosophical Investigations* (New York: Macmillan, 1958), 18.

18. Wittgenstein, *Philosophical Investigations*, 18.

19. Asch and Geller, "Feminism, Bioethics and Genetics."

20. Nancy Press, "Assessing the Expressive Character of Prenatal Testing."

21. Saul Kripke, *Naming and Necessity* (Cambridge, Mass.: Harvard University Press, 1980).

22. Laurence Sterne, *The Life and Opinions of Tristram Shandy, Gentleman* (New York: Penguin, 1998).

23. Marya Schechtman, *The Constitution of Selves* (Ithaca, N.Y.: Cornell University Press, 1996).

24. Hilde Lindemann Nelson, *Damaged Identities, Narrative Repair* (Ithaca, N.Y.: Cornell University Press, 2001).

25. Nora Ellen Groce, *Everyone Here Spoke Sign Language: Hereditary Deafness on Martha' s Vineyard* (Cambridge, Mass.: Harvard University Press, 1988).

26. Bérubé's concern is worth spelling out. Writing about his son, he says

"The danger for children like Jamie does not lie in women's freedom to choose abortion; nor does it lie in prenatal testing. The danger lies in the creation of a society that combines eugenics with enforced fiscal austerity. In such a society, it is quite conceivable that parents who 'choose' to bear disabled children will be seen as selfish or deluded. Among the many things I fear coming to pass in my children's lifetime, I fear this above all: that children like James will eventually be seen as 'luxuries' employers and insurance companies cannot afford, or as 'luxuries' the nation or the planet cannot afford." (Bérubé, *Life as We Know It*, 52).

2

Agency by Proxy

In *The New Yorker* for 27 July 1998, the distinguished British literary critic John Bayley wrote of his forty-five year relationship with his wife, the equally distinguished philosopher and novelist Iris Murdoch.[1] I learned only from this essay's first few pages what has since become widely known—the subject of several books by Bayley, to say nothing of a Miramax film—that Murdoch was suffering from Alzheimer's disease. The news shook me. I had a sudden and sharp recollection of autumn walks in Oxford in the late 1980s, struggling with Murdoch's *The Sovereignty of Good*, its deep suspicion of the "fat, relentless ego" and its (to me) disturbing insistence that the imagination be subject to close interrogation and careful discipline.[2] Her work left me feeling that I had no retreat from the scrutiny of morality, that no place was private enough to escape its judgments, not even my own fantasies. That the person who had with such disciplined imagination of her own so brilliantly explored the complexity and the perniciousness of the ego should now be undergoing its slow effacement struck me as bitterly poignant.

Yet on returning to Bayley's essay, and later reading his books *Elegy for Iris* and *Iris and her Friends*, I didn't find there the same jarring sense of painful irony. Though far from free of anxiety, fear, sadness, and moments of despair, Murdoch, as depicted by her husband, was apparently spared the full ravages this disease can inflict. According to Bayley's account, she did not seem to suffer much from her awareness of what she was losing, the kind of torment Bayley calls the "loss of identity." I find his explanation of her avoidance of this particularly horrible feature of progressive dementia fascinating:

Iris once told me that the question of identity had always puzzled her. In fact, she thought that she herself hardly possessed such a thing, whatever it was. I replied that she must know what it was like to be oneself, even to revel in the consciousness of oneself, as a secret and separate person—a person unknown to any other. She smiled, was amused, and looked uncomprehending.[3]

Just as fascinating, I think, are Bayley's reflections on what Murdoch's illness has done to their relationship:

Life is no longer bringing the pair of us "closer and closer apart," in A.D. Hope's tenderly ambiguous words. Every day, we move closer and closer together. We could not do otherwise. There is a certain comic irony—happily, not darkly comic—that, after more than forty years of our taking our marriage for granted, marriage has decided it is tired of this and is taking a hand in the game. Purposefully, persistently, involuntarily, our marriage is now getting somewhere. It is giving us no choice, and I am glad about that.[4]

Like Bayley, though with less grace, the themes I will explore in this chapter include personal relationships and how they bear on personal identity, as these matters present themselves in the context of serious illness. I'll be interested in how relationship and identity affect agency and the authority to make decisions for others. I'll be aiming to lay at rest—or at least quiet—a somewhat spectral view of persons and their relationships that's been haunting bioethics from its inception as a distinct discourse. My target has been enormously influential practically, and has quite respectable philosophical bona fides. Still, I will argue that it is too insubstantial to accommodate the kinds of complexities latent in real lives and evident in Bayley's accounts of his relationship with Murdoch, and that theoretically it stands not alone, but in the midst of interesting philosophical alternatives.

To put it more plainly, what I'm challenging here is a collection of ideas about human selves and their relationships that has been particularly visible in the development of the theory and practice of making health care decisions for patients incapable of doing so on their own. In broad strokes, these ideas include the following: both metaphysically and morally, human persons are best understood as essentially individuals. Their access to their own mental lives, including their values and preferences, is unique as a matter of the philosophy of mind, and uniquely significant as a matter of the determination of personal identity, and of ethics and social philosophy. While humans are social animals, whose beliefs and assessments are in some large part functions of various and complex social achievements, philosophically these features of our form of life are rather beside the point; despite their dependence on social networks, human selves have highly particular perspectives on the world and what's important about it, and can express distinct, autonomous agency via their own rational deliberation and choice. There is something crucial about each of us that is, as Bayley might say, "secret," "separate," and "unknown."

This individualist view of human identity admits that socially mediated nurturing, training, and education are required for people to develop and exercise their agency. But it also notes that other people persistently threaten and not infrequently hinder agency's free expression, and that may well be what it regards as most morally significant about human relationships—the threats others pose, not the opportunities they create. If the agency of individual persons going about their lawful occasions is thwarted, then what is most distinctively important about persons is disrespected, and the epistemically privileged perspective such people have on their own welfare is disregarded.

Against this image I want to pose and provide at least some motivation for an alternative view of persons and their relationships, suggested by an evocative phrase from an important essay by the philosopher Naomi Scheman, "Individualism and the Objects of Psychology."[5] She writes there that "we are responsible for the meaning of each other's inner lives, that our emotions, beliefs, motivations and so on are what they are because of how they—and we—are related to others in our world—not only those we share a language with, but *those we most intimately share our lives with.*"[6]

What I look to do here, then, is to see whether an alternative vision of personal identity and intimate relationship might be philosophically available and bioethically pertinent. Some of the ideas supporting this vision are at least distantly owing to Wittgenstein, although I will be discussing them as they are handled by more recent thinkers. But first, I want to provide a quick sketch of why the picture I oppose has been so captivating for bioethics. Some of its attraction may well rest on rather general features of the social ideologies regnant in Western democracies, perhaps particularly in the U.S. But I will take a narrower focus and discuss the matter in terms of the explicit agenda of the field.

AUTONOMY'S AMBIGUOUS ASCENDANCY

American bioethics has, in the main, been much taken with the general picture of metaphysical identity and moral significance as essentially individualistic properties, and that probably shouldn't be surprising. For, in addition to whatever it is about American culture that makes "solidarity" seem such a foreign-sounding value, one of bioethics' central concerns has been with individuals immersed in situations in which they are highly vulnerable—sick people, caught up in socially alienating and technically complex systems of health care that may well be benevolently motivated, but that have traditionally been highly paternalistic in the expression of that benevolence. For the latter half of this century, U.S. bioethics and health-related law have been hammering away at health care paternalism, insisting that the patient be seen as a person whose autonomy must be respected, and accordingly, whose informed consent is required to make a health care professional's interventions medicine rather than mayhem. And, at least in the worlds of theory, of courts, classrooms, conferences, and committees, bioethics has scored some notable victories. Virtually everybody talks the language of respect for patient autonomy, from the bioethicists and lawyers who make their living wielding such ideas, to the first-year primary care residents with whom I have worked in Tennessee, Michigan, and New York, most of whom have little inclination for anything that smacks too much of theory.

There is, however, reason to think that bioethics' victories here have been largely notional. Empirical studies tend to indicate that practice is still to a considerable extent driven by values other than respect for the autonomous decision making of individual patients. The Study to Understand Prognosis and Preferences for Outcomes and Risks of Treatment—inevitably known as the SUPPORT study—is the most famous (one might say notorious) of these studies.[7, 8] Concluded in 1995, this five-year, two-phase longitudinal study of several thousand seriously ill patients in five American hospitals revealed that the care of dying patients in the U.S. is a grimmer enterprise than it need be. For example, in the study's first two-year phase, 31 percent of enrolled patients did not want to undergo the trauma of attempted cardiopulmonary resuscitation in the event of heart failure. Slightly fewer than half of their physicians accurately understood this preference. While most of the study participants who ended up dying in the hospital did ultimately manage to get a "do not resuscitate" order, about half the time the order was issued within two days of death, suggesting that careful advance care planning was not the order of the day. Pain control was regarded as poor. And so forth.

On the assumption that the problems revealed by the first phase of the study were largely a matter of poor communication between patients and physicians, SUPPORT's second phase featured an extremely resource-rich intervention designed to get information flowing more freely among health care professionals, patients, and their families. The heart of the intervention was a group of nurses who had been specially trained in ethics and communications. These nurses were exclusively assigned to SUPPORT patients randomized to the interventional arm of the study. It was the nurses' job to initiate reflection and improve communication among patients, family members, and the regular health care team. They promoted advance planning concerning the use of life-extending treatments, documented patients' treatment wishes regarding future care, and tried to improve pain management.

Doctors were also given brief written reports concerning their patients' probabilities of surviving up to six months, their likelihood of severe functional impairment, and their probability of surviving cardiopulmonary resuscitation attempts. Finally, the doctors were also provided with short reports on patients' views about whether they wanted resuscitation attempted should they suffer cardiac arrest, about the severity and frequency of their pain, and about how interested they were in being informed about their medical situations.

All to no avail. The implementation of this extremely expensive intervention, designed by very bright, clinically savvy people, had absolutely no statistically significant effect on the quality of the dying patients' experience, contrasted either against the first phase of the study, or against a group of "control" patients that did not receive the SUPPORT intervention. Patients' views about attempted resuscitation were equally poorly understood by their attending physicians, their pain was just as badly controlled, discussions about reasonable goals of care were held in no more frequent or timely a fashion.

With poor communication demoted as a likely cause of the ethically disturbing practice patterns, it seems, then, that there remains plenty of reason for bioethicists to be concerned about whether the preferences of individual patients are being well respected. Further, both the SUPPORT study, and other studies focusing more directly on decision making for patients too ill to make contemporaneous choices on their own behalf, contain what is perhaps an even more disquieting message. Family members, and other intimates of patients, traditionally relied upon to transmit the preferences and defend the interests of their vulnerable loved ones, don't seem up to the job.

SUPPORT hints at this problem: while family members indicated that half of all patients who could communicate had moderate or severe pain at least half of the time during their last three days of life, they also reported that they *were generally satisfied* with the care their relatives had received—recall that this was care that not only involved inadequate pain control, but also considerable physician confusion about patient preferences and delayed or absent discussion about the medical management of death. On first face, anyway, such satisfied family members hardly look like zealous advocates for their relatives' interests and values.

Even more seriously, perhaps, there is also reason to wonder whether family members are any less confused about what those preferences actually might be than were the SUPPORT physicians. A number of proxy accuracy studies indicate that preferences for treatment are not much better understood by people intimately bonded to patients than they are by physicians. In a *Hastings Center Report* article surveying the relevant empirical literature Linda Emanuel and Ezekiel Emanuel reported that "many studies have indicated that concordance between patient and proxy is far from perfect. The patient's prior wishes and proxy predictions of the patient's prior wishes in circumstances other than the patient's current health overlap only from 33 to 68 percent of the time."[9]

PROXY DECISION MAKING:
CONTENT AND AGENCY

These results set into relief several important features of current discussion and current practice pertaining to proxy decision making. They underscore the threat to their dignity and welfare that vulnerable people face, even within an institution devoted to their care. They weaken confidence in what are widely seen as the primary reasons why close family members have been regarded as "natural proxies" for patients unable to make treatment decisions on their own: if families are not reliable as repositories of zealous advocacy for and discerning insight into the preferences and interests of their members, then they seem disenfranchised as authoritative surrogate decision makers.

The orthodox response to this problem calls for advance planning for health care to become a more explicit matter, with people encouraged to provide their health care professionals with clear and frequently updated statements of their general values and specific treatment preferences, or, at least, formally to authorize family members, or whomever they may prefer, to serve as surrogate health care decision makers should the need arise, after first engaging in the kinds of explicit discussions that should improve the ability of the designated proxy to choose as her principle would have chosen. In the United States, there is federal law in place designed to foster just this sort of outcome.

The orthodoxy has powerful philosophical backing. Trying to make advance care planning based on well-informed and clear patient preferences more pertinent, more prevalent, and more respected can draw for its justification on what Allen Buchanan and Dan Brock call in their highly authoritative book, *Deciding for Others*, "the advance directive principle." The advance directive principle states that "where a clear and bona fide advance directive is available, it is to be followed."[10] That is to say, if a patient can no longer competently form or express her own decisions regarding treatment, and there is a written record of her treatment preferences, or an explicitly named individual whom she has chosen to act in her stead, deference to such a record or person should take precedence over any other way of guiding proxy decision makers—over concern for a patient's best interests, for instance, or the effort to simulate the patient's decision making using a knowledge of the patient's values and of the specific circumstances at hand to judge as the patient would have judged. For in providing an advance directive, the patient is to be understood as exercising her power of self-determination over the course of her treatment, and the exercise of self-determination is greatly prized, both intrinsically and instrumentally.[11]

In articulating and defending the advance directive principle, Buchanan and Brock are taking to a higher degree of sophistication a notion already made influential by previous work, including the early 1980s report of the U. S. President's Commission for the Study of Ethical Problems in Medicine and Biomedical and Behavioral Research.[12] The animating notion is that health care decisions should be made as the patient would make them were she in a position to do so; advance directives give a person a chance to do this, either by specifying particular treatment decisions or particular treatment deciders.

This seems eminently reasonable. But there are a number of difficulties. Some concern such things as the pertinence of written treatment directives, their vagueness or ambiguity. Some concern whether the preferences memorialized in a person's directive are actually the preferences she would have espoused immediately before losing her capacity to make decisions. And some have to do with the way in which explicit advance directives may come to be accorded so much authority that in their absence, other grounds of proxy decision-making authority may not be taken seriously. This last concern is very troubling, given that most people for whom treatment decisions need to be made will not have executed explicit advance directives. It might turn out for such people that their own intimates, the people they may regard as most fitted to make decisions for them, are disenfranchised because they lack the authorization of a legal document naming them as the appropriate proxy. Particularly in cases where a family members' preferred mode of treatment may seem odd to professional health care providers—perhaps a family member is willing for a relative to undergo more pain than is absolutely necessary in order to lengthen life or preserve awareness and hence the ability to relate to those around her—the person most intimate with the patient may be unseated from a decision-making role.[13]

These may, of course, seem to be risks well worth taking in the light of study-supported skepticism about the accuracy of family members' beliefs about patient treatment preferences. If we were to extend to family members a defeasible presumption of proxy decision-making authority even in the face of such skepticism, we would, as the Emanuels see it, be settling for a system that would not honor "the patient's autonomy in treatment choices."[14] I take them to mean that we fail to honor patient autonomy if we don't do our level best to decide the way the patient would decide, and that presumptively relying on family proxies is not anywhere near our level best. But their position may rest on too simple conceptions of the notions crucially in play here.

There are, I suggest, two distinguishable dimensions to the idea "the way the patient would decide." One is the dimension of *content*. Relative to the content dimension, you decide the way the patient would decide if you elect the option that she would have chosen had she been competent to do so. This is what the Emanuels seem to have in mind. The second dimension I will call the dimension of *agency*. Agency I will understand to involve the deliberative perspective from which one assesses options and chooses among them in a way that strives to promote coherence among one's values, plans, and projects. You decide the way a patient would have decided along this dimension to the extent that you reason from the same "deliberative set," seeking coherence among the same values, plans, and projects, as would the patient. Typically, of course, these dimensions of decision making will ride in tandem. But one can imagine them coming apart in contexts where decisions have to be made in someone's behalf by others.

Consider the following scenario, which I will call the Computer Proxy. We are several decades in the future, and treatment decision making across a wide variety of disease-treatment-outcome triads has been extensively studied, and correlated with various demographic markers—age, gender, ethnicity, range of ability, religion, social and economic status, and so forth. As an alternative to decision making by written treatment directives (too blunt, too vague, too ambiguous) or via designated health care proxies (often family members, who too frequently just get it wrong), this demographically based analysis has yielded algorithms that trials show can predict with 99 percent accuracy what a person would have decided were she able to do so.

The Computer Proxy seems to pose a challenge to the advance directive principle: rather than have people try to guess at what their medical fate holds in store for them, or choose unreliable relatives or friends to do the job, just pop the diagnosis, prognosis, and treatment options into the appropriately programmed computer, and the computer will decide "as the patient would have decided."

Would the development of such a program trump the advance directive principle? It seems that if "deciding as the patient decides" is solely a matter of content, it ought to. In fact, with such a device at hand, one might wonder whether we should bother to inflict the difficulties of decision making even on competent patients. But, at least intuitively, there is something that does not love the computer proxy. In discussing this case with a variety of people, I have typically gotten one of two responses. Some people would rather have their decisions made for them by people they count as family, despite the fact that they accept that the computer would be more accurate. Others would like their family proxies to have the computer as a resource, one that would relieve them of at least part of the burden of decision making, but want the final decision to rest in human hands.

I don't claim that these results would necessarily hold up if a valid sample were taken, nor that there is only one clear way to interpret them. However, it does seem to me that they suggest that selecting against the algorithm is a preference we should be able to make sense of. If we can indeed pry apart agency and content, then we may be able to provide a useful gloss on what makes electing the much more fallible human proxy not only intelligible, but reasonable. The suggestion is this: other people may provide us with a form of proxy decision making that, to one degree or another, preserves the dimension of agency. The straightforward sense in which this is true is when they serve at our explicit pleasure. But others may also be well placed and well disposed to reason in a way nourished by and responsive to what we wish to promote, preserve, or aim at—to take up, that is, our deliberative point of view—even if we have not explicitly authorized them to do so. Such people thereby have a source of authority to act as surrogate decision makers apart from their expertise (or otherwise) in constructing the subjunctive preferences of patients not now able to make treatment decisions. The Computer Proxy does not deliberate at all. Rather, it maps demographic information onto treatment options. Hence, despite its superior performance within the dimension of content, it does nothing to preserve agency.

To a considerable extent, the Buchanan-Brock advance directives principle acknowledges the significance of the dimension of agency. Advance directives, they point out, are not merely evidence of what people's preferences might be. They are *expressions* of their preferences, exercises of their agency, "performances that constitute acts of will," and hence have more authority than even well-grounded ideas about what forms of treatment might be in a patient's interest that run counter to the directive.[15] But even though the separable significance of the dimension of agency is noted, the assumption seems to be that a patient's agency can only be exercised by the patient herself absent an explicit authorization.

It is at this point, I think, that the supposition that human selves are fundamentally individual, essentially distinct from all others— "secret," "separate," "unknown"—is close to the surface. There is no in-principle difficulty with my entertaining qualitatively the same preferences concerning your care as you do, for instance. But what is thought to be significant about performances of acts of will is not qualitative identity but numerical identity, or so it seems, and human selves are so constituted that the identity conditions of their mental acts involve essential and necessarily exhaustive reference to particulars that characterize those selves alone. The mere fact, for example, that you and I have lived closely together provides no grounds for thinking that you can exercise my agency on my behalf—not, at least, without my express authorization.

I want to contrast to this view an alternative understanding of agency, one that explicitly allows for the possibility that agency may be shared without explicit authorization, and that appropriately situated people may not only have authority to *interpret,* but also to *change*, the treatment preferences of incompetent patients.

SHARED AGENCY

Buchanan and Brock speak of the execution of an advance directive as an act of will, not merely as evidence of preference, and accord it special authority on that basis. However, the way in which our current acts of will bind our futures is, on Carol Rovane's view, not different in kind from the way in which the undertakings of several selves can express a shared agency. In her book, *The Bounds of Agency*, she notes that what makes the act of will authoritative in the future-regarding case is not that such acts now can causally determine how I will act in the future; holding that position ignores the agency of future states of myself.[16] (Nor, of course, can it determine causally how others will respond to my decisions—that would ignore *their* agency.) What gives a decision its authority, as Rovane sees it, is, so to speak, where it comes from and where it is going. Agents as such possess deliberative points of view, constellations of beliefs and values, and what she refers to as "unifying projects." Such projects require for their planning and execution that an agent deliberate and act so as to strive for "overall rational unity." Overall rational unity denotes a harmony among the agent's beliefs and values achieved via rational operations of thought-weighing evidence, testing for consistency, and so forth. Respecting the agency expressed in an advance directive would, on Rovane's account, involve acknowledging that the unifying project espoused by the competent self embraces the incompetent stage of the self as well. It would involve the belief that the decision was achieved by rationally respectable means.

This view may seem overly rationalist, and too insistent on notions such as "unifying projects" and "overall rational unity" to be plausible, especially in a time whose temper is all for noting the significance of the nonrational, and of caesurae, aporias, and other forms of discontinuity and disunity, both within the self and elsewhere. But from a bioethical perspective that puts such stress on autonomy and competence, it would seem odd to cavil that Rovane is over-privileging the rational element in agency. Nor is she at all inhospitable to disunities—it is an explicit consequence of her position that given unifying projects may not absorb all the resources of a single human, and that hence, distinct, multiple agents may inhere inside, as it were, one human self. But the point I want particularly to stress here is that there is no in-principle barrier in her account to *more* than one human being sharing the same deliberative point of view, striving to make decisions that reflect a shared conception of overall rational unity, centering on a shared unifying project. "There is," she writes,

> no logical or metaphysical reason why there could not be such a joint endeavor that required a plurality of human beings to achieve overall rational unity together . . . we can without any incoherence imagine something like a marital arrangement approximating the ideal of such rational unity. It would be an arrangement in which the partners agreed always to pool all of their information, and always to deliberate jointly from that common pool of information, and always to exert their practical energies together. If two human beings were committed to such a marital arrangement, they would also have to be committed to achieving overall rational unity between them.[17]

If these conditions are met, then agency is sharable without explicit authorization. Or, if you like, the authorization would come, not from a decision or an undertaking, but from an achievement of a shared deliberative point of view.

Of course, the rejoinder will be that this analysis describes at best a notional possibility—no real marriages, partnerships, or friendships are that close. While I don't deny this altogether, it does strike me that certain relationships may approach such a condition, even though asymptotically. Perhaps it is to such a condition that Bayley alludes when he speaks of his marriage as finally "heading somewhere"—in part, perhaps, due to the simplification of Murdoch's own distinctive mental life, but in part also due to Bayley's growing appreciation of the depth of their relationship over the decades in which they shared their lives together. And insofar as relationships characterized by various forms of intimacy approach overall rational unity, relative to particular projects, we might be able to think in terms of degrees of shared agency. This would open a door to seeing how intimates might claim a decision-making authority that is not solely a matter of their accuracy at transmitting a preference, or deducing the implications of a value. This form of authority would stem from the fact that the deliberations of both the principle and the proxy about life and what matters in it had employed similar ideas about facts and values, understood the nuances of those ideas in similar ways, and had used them to reason in similar fashion. A bond of this sort preserves at least some degree of the moral authority we attribute to the patient's own exercise of her agency.

I will later discuss a case where two people have largely shared a deliberative perspective. But as a way to appreciate the significance to our notion of agency of how deliberation goes on, as well as what it achieves, I first will sketch a series of variants on the Computer Proxy case. Recall that in the original case, the computer came up with its marvelously accurate predictions on the basis of demographic information. Imagine a new program, Computer Proxy 2.0: While its predictive powers are no greater than those of the original program, they are predicated not on demographics, but on information more particularly about you as a person—on, say, an analysis of your past patterns of choice, risk-aversion, and so on. Imagine now Computer Proxy 2.1. Again, its ability to produce treatment directives that correspond to yours are no better or worse than the earlier incarnations, but this version works off of a program that explicitly models your particular view of the good, with some sensitivity to how various fact-patterns tend to highlight, or alternately to silence, the practical implications of the various dimensions of your values.

My own sense is that each alteration makes the notion of relying on the computer proxy progressively more inviting, and I'm inclined to attribute that to the computer's more closely modeling not merely the content of a person's preferences, but her agency as well—the characteristic ways in which she develops, understands, ranks, and implements her preferences; at each upgrade, the program more faithfully and fully represents her.

SOCIALLY EXTENDED PERSONHOOD

Computer Proxies 2.0 and 2.1 are fantasies; family and friends are not. To one extent or another, from one situation to another, people who have shared their lives can be in position to model each others' ways of making decisions. But the point I want to make plausible here is not merely that at least some of those who are close to us may be able to engage in practical reasoning in much the same way we do (a sort of qualitative similarity); I also want to take with full seriousness Rovane's idea that our agency can be not just similar but shared.

Another way of appreciating the cogency of the idea of shareable agency is to ally Rovane's conception with so-called "externalism" or "anti-individualist" perspectives in the philosophy of mind. I will consider both the classical externalist position, associated most strongly with Tyler Burge,[18] and then a more recent view called "active externalism," as developed by Andy Clark and David Chalmers.[19]

My approach to these bioethically little-known positions is by way of a philosophical discussion on the nature of persons and their interests familiar to bioethicists, one that has figured seriously in contemporary mainstream discussions of proxy decision making. Neo-Lockean conceptions of personal identity in general, and Derek Parfit's claim that it is not (bivalent) personal identity that matters, but (graded) psychological continuity, in particular, that has struck several thoughtful writers as having interesting implications for proxy decision-making policy.[20] Briefly put, the concern is that understanding personal identity in terms of psychological continuity, or replacing personal identity talk with psychological continuity talk, threatens the authority of advance directives. On some interpretations, simply becoming decisionally incapacitated—the very condition that triggers the applicability of the advance directive—introduces an ontological discontinuity, resulting in there being a numerical distinction between the person making the advance directive and the individual upon whom its instructions will be effected. They are two separate people, not merely different "time slices" of one and the same persisting individual. Others see moderate to severe dementia as calling the preservation of identity into question. For still others, incompetence in general or dementia in particular signals a diminution of the authority of an earlier stage of a self to direct the care of a latter stage, since it is the richness of psychological connections that matters morally.

In their discussion of this problem, Buchanan and Brock suggest that the most troubling variant of the personal identity problem for the advance directive principle really does not involve a rupture in identity. Rather, the toughest case would arise if an apparently "pleasantly demented" person had executed a treatment directive when competent specifying that no life-saving interventions of any sort were to be provided, even in the face of easily treatable illnesses.[21] Rebecca Dresser[22] and Ronald Dworkin[23] have discussed just such a possibility, based on a narrative introduced into the literature by Andrew Firlik.[24] Firlik tells a story about Margo, a woman with Alzheimer's disease, who is very largely dependent on other people, but not so demented that she is without interests or sources of gratification. She is still able to converse with people (although she probably cannot remember who they are, or that she has spoken to them before). She is still able to read mystery novels (although her place in the book skips randomly through the text from day to day). She likes music (which sometimes evokes memories of her dead husband) and painting (although she paints the same simple, peaceful image day after day).

Margo is suffering from a horrible disease, but she seems to be one of the more fortunate of its victims. She has a number of rich interests remaining to her, and in some respects, at least, seems to be having a good life; Firlik speaks of her as "one of the happiest people I have ever known."[25] Now let's add a couple extra features to her story. One is that Margo contracts pneumonia, a disease both easily treatable and potentially lethal. The second is that, when still healthy, she filed an advance directive stating that she wants nothing other than palliative care should she ever succumb to a progressive dementing illness such as Alzheimer's. We can imagine that, prior to the onset of her illness, she always thought of dementia as her personal version of Dante's Ninth Circle. In fact, we can go further and imagine that she anticipated the possibility of *losing precisely this repugnance* as a result of the disease, and dreaded that most of all. So there need be no worry about whether Margo ever anticipated that the actual experience of dementia might not be fairly benign from the perspective of actually having the disease, or whether she had imagined that an easily tolerated and highly effective treatment might not preserve her life. She did; she didn't want any.

The question Dresser raises is whether the views about the significance of life and the conditions of its dignity held by Margo when competent ought automatically take priority over the interests held by the contemporaneous Margo in her comfortable and pleasant, albeit demented, life. On Dresser's view, Margo's current best interests should govern. Ronald Dworkin has offered a much different take on how we should respond to Margo's dementia, one that rides on his notion that there is an important distinction to be drawn among the interests that people have. In his book *Life's Dominion*, he writes:

> Most people think that they . . . have what I shall call critical interests: interests that . . . make their life genuinely better to satisfy, interests they would be mistaken, and genuinely worse off, if they did not recognize. Convictions about what helps to make a life good on the whole are convictions about those more important interests. They represent critical judgments rather than just experiential preferences.[26]

So the issue between Dresser and Dworkin with regard to Margo is just this: when interests based on critical judgments clash with interests based on experiential preferences, which are to be given priority? Dworkin thinks that we should withhold antibiotics from Margo and allow her to die, in keeping with her critical interests; Dresser believes that Margo's experiential interests should prevail and that she should be treated for the pneumonia. Dresser appeals to ideas drawn from Parfit, arguing that demented Margo may not be the same person—or "enough" of the same person—for the earlier critical interests to be applicable to the instant decision, although she does not rest her case fully on his notion of personal identity. Dworkin relies on the fact that critical interests play a crucially important normative role in the career of a person. We value these interests because they are important; they are not important simply because we value them. They outline our best, most reflective judgments about the structure of our lives, about wherein lies our integrity as persons.

Dresser argues that, in insisting that critical interests be dispositive, we are losing sight of the Margo before us; she becomes a "Missing Person," lost in a haze of theory. Dworkin might reasonably reply that it is Dresser who has lost sight of Margo. In focusing on her condition at the present moment, she has neglected Margo as a person, the significance of whose life transcends the present moment. Rather than recognizing her life as a richly textured story, in which the meaning of what is presently going on must be seen against the background of all that has gone before it, she has reduced Margo to a disconnected episode, plucked out of a bundle of fleeting sensations.

But if there is a temporal dimension to the significance of our lives that Dresser underplays, there is, I think, an interpersonal dimension to that significance that Dworkin misses. Although he insists that our critical interests retain their significance even after we lose the ability to appreciate them, or to tend to their maintenance and reshaping, he seems to assume, quite without argument, that once a person permanently loses her decision-making capacity, her critical interests are fixed in stone—all that others can do is to try to determine what they are, and then respect them.

Let's imagine that Margo did not file an advanced directive, but did have a so-called natural proxy—her daughter, Ann. On both Dresser's and Dworkin's view, Ann's job is purely hermeneutic. Dworkin would see Ann's job as interpreting how the various choices facing Margo relate to her enduring critical interests; for Dresser, the interpretive task would be to determine and act in accordance with Margo's best experiential interests. But I want to suggest that Ann may well face a constructive as well as a hermeneutical job; she may be in a position to make decisions that reflect an evolution of Margo's critical interests, one that may involve Margo in a kind of moral redefinition.

Here's an argument for this piece of heterodoxy. Dworkin's view that Margo's critical interests are fixed in stone once she becomes demented seems to make most theoretical sense when viewed as a version of what's sometimes called "internalism" (or, interestingly, "individualism") in the philosophy of mind. On an individualist view, the meaning of what occurs in our minds can be understood wholly in terms of properties or events that happen altogether in the individual herself. When the relevant internal properties cease, some mental contents just cease with them. Critical interests endure—indeed, they may even survive death—but the mechanism of forming and changing them, involving reflection, deliberation, agency, is inoperable.

Since the work of Saul Kripke and other philosophers of language writing in the early 1970s, there's reason to think such a view of our mental lives leaves rather too much up to us as individuals.[27] Suppose that part of the contents of Ronald Dworkin's mind can be represented accurately by the following sentence: "Jane Austen is the author of *Sense and Sensibilia.*" (We see that he's made a little mistake here.) One puzzle is figuring out how the words "Jane Austen" manage to pick out that woman, Jane Austen herself. A familiar view is that Dworkin possesses a set of beliefs, inside his own head, as it were, that he associates with the name, and which succeed in uniquely specifying that very woman, and no one else. Now this might seem plausible if Dworkin's beliefs about Austen include such descriptions as "the currently most famous female Regency novelist," or "the woman who in the early 19th century created the character Emma." But suppose he associates the name with such beliefs as "the author of 'Three Ways of Spilling Ink,'" or "an Oxford don renowned for her interest in the *Oxford English Dictionary.*" Then it seems natural to say that he has a lot of false beliefs about Jane Austen. But it remains the case that his false beliefs are about Miss Austen, that he somehow is able to refer to her despite the false beliefs. This suggests that beliefs do not play the role in securing reference that the familiar view claims.

In fact, even if Dworkin has nothing but true beliefs about Jane Austen, it still seems unlikely that the belief view tells the right story about how the contents of his mind connect to the extra-mental world. If the meaning of a name is what secures its reference, it would seem that Dworkin's individuating beliefs about Austen would have to be part of the meaning of the name, and if this is the case, it becomes a necessary truth that "Jane Austen wrote the novel *Emma.*" But surely this must be wrong. It is perfectly possible—although luckily, not actual—that, about that very woman, it was not true that she wrote any books at all. She might have died as a child. That circumstance would have prevented her from being a famous author, but not from being Jane Austen.[28]

These are, of course, well-worn considerations by now that have generated their countermoves in turn. But at least it can be said that there is a respectable alternative to a view of how names denote, and of what our minds are stocked with. This is the anti-individualist view, and it understands our ability to refer to the world, not as due to "meanings" analytically linked with words, but rather in virtue of actual historical-causal relationships between what goes on in our mental or verbal use of language and features of the world that surrounds us.[29] Now I want to suggest how a generally anti-individualist view of the mind might transform our—or at least Dworkin's—views about critical interests and how they grow.

Let's suppose that Margo has not only a devoted daughter, but a religion to which she was equally devoted. She was, we will say, a committed member of the Jehovah's Witnesses. Suppose further that the disease she develops in the course of her apparently pleasant dementia requires blood transfusions, not merely antibiotics. I'm confident that Dworkin would find this yet another strong reason to let Margo die, since fidelity to her deepest religious commitments must count as a critical interest if anything does.

But now let's add yet another complication to Margo's story. Suppose that after much reflection and prayerful attention to the matter, the Witnesses have decided that the traditional position on blood transfusion was based on a misreading of the relevant Scripture, and hence, after Margo becomes demented, the doctrine changes. Now, since Margo's commitment to this doctrine was a matter of Church discipline, and not something she affirmed on her own authority as an biblical exegete, it seems at least plausible to hold that one of her critical interests has changed, and not as a result of anything that is going on within her own mind, as it were. If so, it seems that changes in the world can, quite on their own, change the structure of a person's critical interests, even if that person is not in a position to endorse the change explicitly. Critical interests "ain't in the head," to borrow a phrase of Hilary Putnam's. And if this conclusion is reasonable, it would seem that the role of proxy decision makers needs to be understood differently. Their job is not simply to report or even simply to *discern* the patient's interests: it may well be to *evolve* them as well.

To appreciate this point further, consider another variant of Margo's case. Before the onset of Margo's illness, let us suppose, she and Ann had often discussed her special antipathy to dementia, a view Ann shared. However, since Margo developed Alzheimer's disease, Ann has changed her own views, in no small part as a result of caring for, and spending time with, her mother. Ann's shift in view is also due to her continuing religious and ethical reflections. She now thinks that their earlier abhorrence was hyper-rationalistic, too dualistic, not sufficiently sensitive to the importance of embodiment in the religious tradition they both shared. An important critical interest of Ann's— her views about what makes life worth living—has changed. As a result, she no longer thinks that the pneumonia should be allowed to carry her mother off. But if she authorizes the antibiotics, isn't that an abuse of her proxy authority? I think this is far less clear than standard accounts of proxy authority would suggest. Ann's changing views about the significance of a highly cognitive life may occasion a change in the mother's interests about these matters as well, just as occurred in the Jehovah's Witness variation on this story.

Suppose, for example, Margo's views about dementia had been forged in conversation and joint reflection with Ann, and were supported in part by Margo's confidence in Ann's good moral judgment. In such a situation it seems reasonable to think that Margo and Ann may have shared a deliberative point of view on this matter, and that Margo's relevant critical interests have changed with her daughter's moral reexamination of the issues.

This analysis chimes nicely with Rovane's suggestion that agency may be shared. It also is comparable with Clark and Chalmer's "active externalism."[30] On their view, if we allow that people can have beliefs apart from those immediately occurrent to them—if, that is, we allow what are called dispositional beliefs—we have no good reason to deny that an individual may have beliefs stored "outside their skin." Clark and Chalmers motivate this view by discussing the case of Inga and Otto, both of whom are seeking out New York City's Museum of Modern Art. Inga has heard about an exposition she'd like to attend, reflects for a moment on where the museum is, and then proceeds to 53rd Street. However, like Ms. Murdoch and Margo, Otto suffers from Alzheimer's disease, and accordingly, he cannot simply reflect on where the museum is, as Inga does, and reliably recall the location. He relies on a notebook, which he carries around with him where ever he goes. "Today, Otto hears about the exposition at the Museum of Modern Art, and decides to go see it. He consults his notebook, which says that the museum is on 53rd Street, so he walks to 53rd Street and goes into the museum."[31]

"Clearly," say Clark and Chalmers, "Otto walked to 53rd Street because he wanted to go to the museum and he believed that the museum was on 53rd Street."[32] The information in his belief just happens to be located not in his brain, but on the other side of his skin. If, however, we deny on such grounds that he has the belief even before he consulted his notebook, we must deny that Inga had her belief before she consulted her memory. The features that distinguish the ways Inga and Otto retrieve the relevant information are, Clark and Chalmers claim, superficial. The fundamental features of beliefs— their role in the explanation of action—"mirror each other precisely" in the two cases. The fact that Inga's mode of access to the information that she needs may differ in some phenomenological characteristics, that hers is "direct," his "perceptually mediated," seems beside the point. If, for instance, Inga's way of recalling where the museum is takes the form of seeming to see the address written in green letters hanging in the middle of her visual field, we might be surprised, but we wouldn't say that she lacked the relevant belief. What is crucial is that the information be accessible and reliable, not whether it is stored in brains or in notebooks.

What is particularly on the present point is the moral Clark and Chalmers derive from their view. Like Rovane, they see no in-principle reason why a person's mental states might not be in part constituted by the states of other thinkers—"unusually interdependent couples," as they call them—and indeed allow that one's "history of past endorsements" might well determine what one knows or believes.

These externalist arguments recall Scheman's words about the unusually interdependent couple in our own example: Ann, the person with whom Margo has "intimately shared her life," "shares the responsibility for the content of her mental life." Margo and her daughter are engaged in a relationship close enough so that their relevant projects closely overlap and their rational points of view encompass very similar beliefs and values, à la Rovane. Margo has depended on Ann to help form and maintain her beliefs, and Ann has been trustworthy, reliable, and accessible, satisfying the conditions for "socially extended cognition" specified by Clark and Chalmers.

SOCIALLY EXTENDED PERSONS AND POLICY

The work of Rovane and of externalist philosophers of mind demonstrates that there are imaginable and defensible conceptions of persons and their relationships that are alternatives to the standard individualist pictures, alternatives that may have implications for proxy decision making in health care. The philosophical motivations for these ideas have only been roughed out here, but rather than develop them further, I want to conclude by discussing some concrete implications of this alternative view of persons, their relationships, and their agency, for day-to-day clinical practice.

At least one policy implication seems to emerge fairly plainly: namely, that family decision making—or more precisely, decision making by bonded intimates—should be the default setting for making health care decisions for those unable to do so on their own, with advance directives as a backdrop for those with no (reliable) intimates or, perhaps, with idiosyncratic preferences. The analyses considered here strongly suggest that this idea should be more closely examined than it has been to date. Admittedly, these arguments cannot themselves secure the case for adopting something closer to a probate law model for proxy health care decision making. We need further empirical inquiry into how health care decisions actually get made, what the role of intimates really is in such decision making, and how satisfactory the result seems to be. There is a considerable amount of suspicion about families around today, no doubt much of it well-founded. Precisely how much suspicion is appropriate, though, is I think still an open question, and how we should revise the proxy decision making mechanisms currently in place has at least something to do with how we answer it.

There is a related, yet deeper point. It is, I think, not all together inaccurate to say that bioethics has tried hard to honor the plural and diverse sources of value, ideas of the good, and risk budgets that different patients present. A liberal interpretation of the respect for autonomy principle, a notion that carries with it a stress on the moral significance of selves considered in the most crucial ways as isolated, has been its main tool in doing so. But, as is commonly claimed in general critiques of liberalism, the conceit that liberal principles and methods provide a fully neutral deliberative perspective may involve an element of self-deception, or at best, be useful only in part. Rather than truly promoting pluralism in medicine, bioethics may simply have rather introduced another distinctive conception of what it is for persons to live well and to choose well, one as remote from many patients' lives as is the benevolent authoritarianism of the traditional hospital.

Between enduring medical paternalism and the sort of individualistic legalism that bioethics has injected into the mix, more particular views of what is good, and of how humans are related one to another, may find themselves squeezed out. Joanne Lynn, a physician-ethicist with tremendous experience with dying patients, has suggested in conversation that what drives people hardest in such circumstances is the desire to be "good," to get it "right." Health care facilities can be such total institutions that patients and their families find themselves looking to the values current in those settings, rather than to their own most important traditions, beliefs, and practices, for guidance in how to be a good patient or family member, how to suffer well, how to die well, or how to let someone die well. Bioethicists have typically been sensitive to how the world of the clinic might alienate people from their own deepest sources of direction and consolation. Unfortunately, bioethicists have been less sensitive to the impact of their own work on patients and their intimates. What might seem the rather abstract enterprise of trying to put into play a richer array of ideas about the metaphysical character of human selves may make something quite concrete plainer to bioethicists—their own complicity in rendering the clinic a foreign and forbidding place.[33]

NOTES

1. John Bayley, "Elegy for Iris," *The New Yorker* 74, no. 21 (1998): 45–61. Bayley's essay occurs in a much expanded form as *Elegy for Iris* (New York: St. Martin's Press, 2000). I discuss this book in "A Reserve Deep and Natural," in *Contemporary Gerontology* 8, no. 4 (2002).
2. Iris Murdoch, *The Sovereignty of Good* (London and New York: Routledge and Kegan Paul, 1970).
3. Bayley, "Elegy," 56.
4. Bayley, "Elegy," 61.
5. Naomi Scheman, "Individualism and the Objects of Psychology," in her *Engenderings* (New York: Routledge, 1993).
6. Scheman, "Individualism," 52. The stress is added.
7. SUPPORT Principle Investigators, "A Controlled Trial to Improve Care for Seriously Ill Hospitalized Patients," *Journal of the American Medical Association* 274 (1995): 1591–98.
8. Ellen H. Moskowitz and James Lindemann Nelson, "The Best Laid Plans," in "Dying Well in the Hospital: The Lessons of SUPPORT," Special Supplement, *Hastings Center Report* 25, no. 6 (1995): S3–S6.
9. Linda Emanuel and Ezekiel Emanuel, "Decisionmaking at the End of Life: Guided by Communities of Patients," *Hastings Center Report* 23, no. 5 (1993): 7.

10. Allen Buchanan and Dan Brock, *Deciding for Others* (Cambridge: Cambridge University Press, 1990), 95.

11. Buchanan and Brock, *Deciding*, 98.

12. U.S. President's Commission for the Study of Ethical Problems in Medicine and Biomedical and Behavioral Research, *Making Health Care Decisions* (Washington, D.C.: U.S. Government Printing Office, 1982).

13. For a discussion of just such a case, see Hilde Lindemann Nelson and James Lindemann Nelson, *The Patient in the Family* (New York: Routledge, 1995), 224ff.

14. Emanuel and Emanuel, "Decisionmaking," 8.

15. Buchanan and Brock, *Deciding for Others*, 97.

16. Carol A. Rovane, *The Bounds of Agency* (Princeton, N.J.: Princeton University Press, 1998).

17. Rovane, *Bounds of Agency*, 141.

18. Tyler Burge, "Individualism and the Mental," *Midwest Studies in Philosophy* 4 (1979): 73–121.

19. Andrew Clark and David Chalmers, "The Extended Mind," *Analysis* 58 (1998): 7–19.

20. Derek Parfit, *Reasons and Persons* (Oxford: Oxford University Press, 1984).

21. Buchanan and Brock, *Deciding for Others*, 188.

22. Rebecca Dresser, "Missing Persons: Legal Perceptions of Incompetent Patients," *Rutgers Law Review* 46 (1994): 609–719.

23. Ronald Dworkin, *Life's Dominion* (New York: Alfred A. Knopf, 1993).

24. Andrew Firlik, "Margo's Logo," *Journal of the American Medical Association* 265 (1991): 201.

25. Firlik, "Margo's Logo," 201.

26. Dworkin, *Life's Dominion*, 201–202.

27. See Saul Kripke, *Naming and Necessity* (Cambridge, Mass.: Harvard University Press, 1980).

28. An earlier version of the same argument appears in James Lindemann Nelson, "Preferences and Other Sources of Family Decisionmaking Authority," *Journal of Law, Medicine and Ethics* 23 (1995): 144–48.

29. Burge, "Individualism and the Mental."

30. Clark and Chalmers, "Extended Mind."

31. Clark and Chalmers, "Extended Mind," 12–13.

32. Clark and Chalmers, "Extended Mind," 13.

33. For a learned and searching discussion of the notion that proxy decision making may be of much greater interest to bioethicists than to patients, see Carl Schneider, *The Practice of Autonomy* (Oxford: Oxford University Press, 1998).

3

Just Expectations
Family Caregivers, Practical Identities, and Social Justice in the Provision of Health Care

For some decades now, dampening the explosive growth of health care costs has been a major policy priority, both in the United States and around the world. While the mid-to-late 1990s cycle of economic expansion in the U.S. significantly tempered the rate at which health care expenditures had been eating up the gross domestic product, costs in this area always were dynamic, fueled by the wide dissemination of new and very expensive technologies. As of this writing, health care spending has resumed its voracious attack on personal, corporate, state, and national budgets.[1]

Not that the health care industry ever put its faith solely in the hope of permanent economic boom. Another key though stealthy force moderating the dizzying upward spiral of health care costs that characterized the 1980s and early 1990s was a sort of semi-voluntary conscription of unpaid health care workers, who generally lacked any professional training for their tasks. This new "draft" has largely escaped attention because of just who was being pressed into service. Responsibilities were shifted from professional caregivers working in hospitals and other such sites, to untrained, ill-experienced, and uncompensated *care-giving relatives* whose work largely takes place at home. Ironically enough, this trend has been coupled with a reduction of home-care benefits available through insurers or public programs.[2]

There is every reason to think that growing reliance on family caregivers will continue to be an attractive tactic. Increasingly complex forms of health care technologies are being more-or-less adapted to home use, and the price remains right. Spouses, parents, and children are cheap compared to RNs or respiratory technicians, and advanced health care technologies can now be directed and monitored remotely, via "telemedicine," speeding the process of turning homes into faux hospitals, and those who live there into health care professionals manqué.[3]

It will be interesting, to say no more, to see how the quality of patient care stands up to this progressive deprofessionalization of health care provision. Diverting responsibilities for patient well-being from highly trained and experienced professionals, who have tolerably clear role-related limits on the extent of the services they are supposed to provide, to an amateur population, often otherwise employed, and with no clear and socially recognized limits to their responsibilities, looks very much like a bad sort of health care rationing. While it does not require that any particular medical service be denied, or any special population be excluded (except, perhaps, those who lack families)—thus avoiding the most visible and controversial forms of rationing—deprofessionalizing the health care work force achieves cost savings at the risk of a more generally distributed dilution of the quality of care available to patients. As a public policy, this shift is close to covert; it is little noted or discussed even by health policy analysts or bioethicists.

Nor are the consequences for family members, pressed into intense, prolonged caregiving roles, likely to be benign. In a recent discussion of the increased role of informal caregivers in the new health economy, Carol Levine—who, as will be shown, has reason to know—summed the matter up bleakly: "Individuals and families will be under increased pressure to pay more direct costs; families will be expected to provide more hands on, often technologically complex care; undertake greater burdens for longer times; and forego more educational, career and social opportunities."[4]

The question of possibly decreased quality of care for patients (particularly if seen as a form of rationing) and questions concerning the "increased pressures" on caregiving individuals and families raise theoretical issues in our understanding of distributive justice that have been largely overlooked by bioethicists. I will focus on the impact of these changes on care providers, in part because the philosophical problems there are particularly fascinating. Surely, it is only the fact that informal caregivers are typically family members that explains why they are dragooned into unpaid and intensive labor with only the faintest whimpers of protest; even in a culture with a notoriously spotty record of respect for women and people identified with ethnic or racial minorities, the notion that any other group could be expected to take on such tasks free of charge is not credible. At the same time, at least some family caregivers who shoulder extreme burdens apparently find great value in the provision of hands-on care to those they love, and they are reluctant to turn to whatever alternative sources of care might still be available. Despite some recent attention to the ethical character of intimate associations, we still lack fully mature accounts of what societies may justly expect of families, and of what family members may justly expect of each other. In what follows, I aim to contribute to the development of such an account, and to trace out some implications bearing on whether the "impressment" of families into more, and more intensive, health care responsibilities can be defended.

ARE FAMILIES BEING UNJUSTLY DONE BY?

Is it consistent with a reasonable account of distributive justice to constrain health care costs by establishing policies that transfer prolonged or intensive health care responsibilities from professionals to family members? This is a complicated question, in part because the trend has not resulted from some central planning agency that might reasonably be held accountable for the systematic effects of its decisions—in this respect, the "conscription" metaphor employed earlier is misleading. The migration of increasingly burdensome health care responsibilities from professionals to family members is a function of many decisions made by federal and state governments, by different private insurers, and, perhaps, even by those insurance consumers who have some measure of realistic choice about the kind of coverage to elect. This ambiguity about agency makes it tougher to determine who bears what responsibility for any resulting harms. It hardly seems plausible that *any* reliance on family for *any* amount or kind of care constitutes an injustice, and so decisions tending to contribute to this trend incrementally may seem more or less innocent.

Allowing that it is appropriate to expect families to sacrifice to at least some extent for their needy members introduces what I think is the most vexing complication. Getting clear about the justice of this kind of deprofessionalization of health care provision is caught up with the question of what family members are entitled to expect of one another, and of what kinds of contributions to social goals such expectations license. To see why this is a tough job, consider the currently leading understandings of distributive justice. Philosophical reflection about distributive justice is often depicted as a matter of discovering and motivating ways of allocating the benefits and burdens

involved in social life in ways that respect some special moral character that human beings are thought to have. In leading forms of contemporary theory, the special character is often indicated with notions like
"inviolability" or "separateness." This is of course the case in liber-
tarian theories, but is also true square in theory's mainstream. John
Rawls is fond of both notions; inadequate respect for the "distinction
between persons"[5] is at the heart of his objection to utilitarian allocation schemes, and, in one of his memorable ringing phrases, he writes
that "each person has an inviolability founded on justice that even the
welfare of society as a whole cannot override."[6] Justice, then, is
thought to involve considering people as individuals with certain
moral prerogatives that must be respected, even if doing so should
make everyone worse off than they otherwise would be.

Think of persons as members of a large, "impersonal" social
arrangement, in which the exploitation of variously marginalized
groups and individuals endures, and the intuitive appeal of notions
such as separateness and inviolability may seem compelling. Think of
persons as members of families in which exploitation, while surely
present, often goes hand in glove with affirmation, caring, and love,
and the appeal flags. Insofar as intimacy is an important good, we have
reason to want it to flourish. It hasn't much chance of doing so in settings where distinctness or separateness are the primary values. The
relationships between members of tolerably intimate families are significantly different in morally important ways from those between
people qua citizens of a state, or qua economic agents in a market-
place.

In reasonably well-functioning families, people will generally find
something more than opportunities to amuse or aggrandize themselves
through arms-length interchanges with similarly motivated others.
Such families are places where our very selves are, in important ways,
formed, sustained, and shared. Individual interests abound in families,
but so do shared interests, and even what might be called the interests
of the family as a whole.[7] Acknowledging that such shared and inter-
defined interests are often importantly characteristic of families does
not require taking an overly roseate view of families as homogenous
and ideal havens. While we may find ourselves, for example,
espousing certain values simply because other family members do,
this hardly excludes our also having distinct and oftentimes conflicting
interests.[8] But the significance of such shared interests as there may
be does make trouble for conceptions of distributive justice that are

predicated on the primary significance of individuality and distinctness to clarify who is indebted to whom for what.

The theoretical emphasis on the "distinctness of persons" is not the only problem in sorting out what family members do and do not owe to each other. Just as you don't have to be a communitarian to acknowledge morally relevant differences between personal relations qua citizen and personal relations qua family member, neither do you have to be a moral particularist to allow that families are rife with different, numerous, and fine-grained morally relevant features. Families tend to endure over significant periods of time, involve people in strong emotions, and play important and varied roles in how people understand themselves and others. The patterns of feeling and action, of duties and of disappointment, and of what goes beyond both duty and disappointment and yet bears on how claims should be sorted out, can differ from relationship to relationship within a family, from time to time within one family,[9] and certainly from family to family. To know, for example, whether some assignment of burdens and benefits is morally defensible, one is going to have to know a good deal about the particular family under consideration.

Despite these difficulties, I want to argue that the shift of health care responsibilities to families does raise questions of justice that are both deeply serious and potentially tractable. There are features of families that make treating them as a standing reserve of labor for the health care system morally problematic.

My argument for this conclusion has two stages. First, I want to call attention to some specific and serious kinds of vulnerability that families generally have to the ongoing shifts in how we apportion health care responsibilities. Second, I will argue that these vulnerabilities are not merely private misfortunes, but are salient from the point of view of distributive justice; there is good reason to see the community as having a duty to deploy its resources to avoid, or at least ameliorate, the harms associated with intensive or prolonged family provision of health care.

THREE THREATS TO FAMILIES

I'll use three considerations to set in relief what is at stake for families in current trends in health care delivery. The first is their *propensity for exploitation*. This particular vulnerability follows fairly directly from the ways in which family members in many instances do not regard their own interests as altogether distinct from their relatives'. Families are not altogether outside what classic theorists such as Hume called the "circumstances of justice": like all human communities, they are composed of people roughly equally vulnerable to fate and to each other, confronting at least moderate scarcity with respect to at least some of what is valued. But they often exist also within "circumstances of intimacy," where caring for, and identification with, other members replaces mutual indifference as a basic motivation.

A nation, for example, might come to the reasonable conclusion that supplying the resources needed to satisfy certain citizens' needs was an unreasonable or even flatly unjust drain on the common pool. Having decided that it need not or even ought not meet such needs, a nation might, in fact, simply let them go unmet; charity (or shame), although they may play some role in public policy, are not overwhelmingly strong motivators. Families might confront similar situations and engage in analogous reasoning leading to the same conclusion. Some of its members may have needs that are simply too great for others to be expected to fulfill. But there are also considerations apart from justice—considerations of love, to take a prominent example—that may lead families, or individuals within families, to provide care over and above what could be expected of them as a matter of justice. This inclination to supererogation makes families prime targets for exploitation.[10]

The second consideration highlights an important feature of the kind of risk that families face. In supplying care that is prolonged and intensive, family members can put in harm's way what I will call (following Christine Korsgaard) their *practical identities*. A practical identity is "a description under which you find your life to be worth living and your actions to be worth undertaking."[11] Korsgaard speaks of people having a "jumble" of such identities ("a human being, a woman or a man, an adherent of a certain religion, a member of an ethnic group, a member of a certain profession, someone's lover or friend . . ."), and regards those identities as providing reasons and obligations: "Your reasons express your identity, your nature; your obligations spring from what that identity forbids."[12]

Some practical identities seem to make more central contributions to our overall sense of self than others; some are more inextricably caught up with our convictions about the worthwhileness of our lives and actions. Further, our grasp on any of our practical identities is surely contingent; misadventure and mortality can take them all away. However, when human agency is involved in wrenching away cherished practical identities from us, the agents are at least presumptively culpable, as they would be for intentionally or negligently causing any serious harm.

Reflecting on the importance of practical identities is on point because the kind of intensive caregiving increasingly demanded of families is not merely a matter of shifting resources from one area of an organization's endeavors to another. Rather, it is very likely to involve a restructuring of people's most basic projects—those activities that are deeply implicated in some of the most fundamental and personally significant ways that people identify themselves. A person's ability to take on and maintain an identity as, say, a breadwinner, a professional, a student, or even a spouse may be impaired or blocked. Sufficiently burdensome caregiving requirements also threaten to harm the character of the family itself, and its ability to discharge competently a central function: nurturing those capacities required for people to take on and pursue their practical identities.

This is clearly the case for children being brought up in families: a family unable to foster the ability of its young to form practical identities, whether due to providing intensive health care or for any other reason, is truly dysfunctional. But it's not just the young who are vulnerable; a family's adults, too, depend on each other to maintain their practical identities. Families typically provide many of the crucial material and expressive resources that enable people to form, consider, endorse, revise, and live out their conceptions of themselves. The significance of practical identities reflects the extent to which people, even in close, interdependent, and intimate families, have distinct identities and projects. Indeed, reflection on practical identities calls attention to the way in which families actually contribute in important ways to the distinctiveness of their members.

The third consideration I want to examine is the tendency of families to *embody patterns of injustice*, and for that tendency to be exacerbated by increased caregiving demands. Families are hardly immune from objectionable uses of gender and age as the basis for assigning duties and benefits to their members. The shift of health care responsibilities from professional to intimate realms threatens to further entrench these biases. Women continue to be assigned primary caregiving tasks to a grossly disproportionate degree, rendering them especially prone to further exploitation in circumstances that involve prolonged or intensive caregiving for family members.[13] As women are typically the "least well off" in families when it comes to having discretionary time and energy after responsibilities at home and in the workplace, social practices that make them still worse off in these respects are particularly suspicious.

While all these considerations will figure in the development of my position, I will concentrate on harm to practical identities, in part because it provides ways of thinking about the relationships between "distinctness" and the forms of value characteristic of intimate associations, and in part because gender and generational justice issues in families can be vividly appreciated by deploying the notion of practical identities; oppression can be understood in terms of the links between the practical identities out of which goals and values emerge, and the social practices that constrict a person's ability to form, pursue, and modify those identities.[14]

THE SOCIAL CONSTRUCTION OF FAMILY CAREGIVING, AND THE CONSTRICTION OF PRACTICAL IDENTITIES

In a pair of remarkable articles, Carol Levine has vividly illustrated ways in which these considerations can play themselves out in families confronting serious health care problems. In her *New England Journal of Medicine* "Sounding Board" essay, "The Loneliness of the Long-Term Care Giver," Levine writes of nearly a decade's experience of being a family care giver to her husband, gravely injured in a car accident early in 1990.[15] She tells us of her nightmares of disconnections and strained connections with the health care system, nightmares that have haunted her awake, as well as asleep. Despite the fact that she is herself a distinguished bioethicist and health policy analyst, it took Levine years to appreciate that her nightmares stemmed not from any inadequacy of her own, but from a "system" that is decidedly unsystematic, and badly out of order to boot. A chilling sentence occurs early in the essay: "During my nine year odyssey, I stopped being a wife and became a family care giver."[16] What is perhaps most striking about this radical shift in one of Levine's central practical identities is that she does *not* link it to the pervasive changes in her profoundly disabled husband, but rather to how *she herself* has been reconfigured by the set of social practices and understandings with which the health care system (and the broader society in which it is nestled) responds to the chronically ill and those with whom their lives are most closely entwined.

During the weeks of her husband's ICU stay, Levine reports that she remained a wife, treated with "kindness and concern." Then came something of a liminal period, when her husband's life was no longer in immediate danger, and she effectively disappeared from the attention of his professional caregivers. When the extent and permanence of her husband's disabilities became clear, she reemerged into view, but under a decidedly different aspect. She was now only the manager and the hands-on provider of his care. During her husband's stay in a rehabilitation facility ("boot camp for care givers," Levine labels it) she was initiated into her new role—the performer of "an unrelieved series of nasty chores," expected to impoverish herself to procure Medicaid funding for the homecare needed by her husband. One anecdote is particularly telling: "A nurse stuck my husband's soiled sweat pants under my nose and said, 'Take these away. Laundry is your job.' A woman whose husband had been at the same facility later told me the same story—different nurse."[17]

Mr. Levine was sent home from rehab a poorly treated, poorly diagnosed man, profoundly physically handicapped, cognitively challenged, emotionally labile—"not the same person in any sense." And, in at least some important senses, neither was Ms. Levine.

I have lingered on this difficult story because it powerfully shows how deeply the experience of chronic illness and disability can penetrate the lives not solely of patients, but also of those intimately engaged with them. It is not hyperbolic to claim that the Levines' story indicates how the current social arrangement for providing care to those with serious and chronic illnesses and disabilities can be life threatening for family caregivers, in a biographic, if not a biological sense. The story makes it plain just how relatives and other bonded intimates pressed into extensive caregiving responsibilities must put the persistence of their central practical identities at risk. It is worth underscoring that this damage is caused not by the flow of funding (although that is surely crucial), but by the way in which family caregivers are portrayed by the health care system with which they interact. In a companion article published in *Ms.*, Levine gives another, more gender-specific, illustration of disparaging attitudes:

> When my husband's prognosis became clear, and the long future stretched ahead of us, I looked for help. None was forthcoming. Even more appalling, the most judgmental responses came from women— nurses and social workers. Some nurses, admittedly overworked, were so resentful of my continuing to work [in her "outside" job] and failing to relieve them of their duties that I had to hire a "companion" to be with

my husband in the rehab center until I arrived each day at 4 P.M. to feed him. When he screamed for help (regularly) or was uncooperative (even more frequently), I was blamed.[18]

While Levine was having to bear the system's scorn, the spouse of another patient, who visited with fanfare and flowers every few evenings, was being effusively greeted by the nurses. This patient was a woman; her "wonderful" spouse, a man. When Levine noted the discrepancy, she was told by a nurse, "You don't realize how rare it is for men to stay involved."[19]

Levine's articles distinctively highlight two interrelated dimensions of the damage family caregivers face. One of these dimensions is material: family caregivers do not generally command the financial resources to enable them to both care for their relative and maintain and develop the range of practical identities they previously enjoyed. The other is expressive: family caregivers—particular women—are caught up in socially enacted narratives that tend to silence the diversity of caregiver identities and emplot them as caregivers plain and simple.[20]

There is nothing fundamentally idiosyncratic about Levine's experience. For example, in the United Hospital Fund of New York's recent Special Report, *Rough Crossings: Family Caregivers' Odysseys through the Health Care System*, the derangement of practical identities caused by family provided health care is plain in case after case.[21] Consider the story of Theresa and Robert Smith and their eighteen-year-old daughter Jill, for instance. Jill was struck by a delivery van and suffered severe neurological trauma. She remained in a coma for two weeks, and when she emerged, she was unable to speak or control her limbs, bladder, or bowels. Jill needed to be strapped into her bed so that she wouldn't injure herself. When inpatient insurance ran out after the second month, Theresa and Robert decided to care for Jill at home, finding themselves immediately caught up in a grueling caregiving practice that seemed to have no end. They campaigned tirelessly for a range of services for their daughter, including physical, occupational, and speech therapy, nursing care and equipment. They also tried to secure good home health aides to help care for Jill. Taking all this on required significant and systematic changes in the Smiths' lives. Theresa cut her out-of-the-home job to part time, devoting the rest of her day to Jill's needs, including overseeing the stream of home attendants who passed into, and then quickly out of, their lives. In the discussion of this case, we read:

Robert received little attention from his wife. During evening meals, which were usually take-out, she would engage him in decisions about Jill's care, and conflict often erupted. After a long day at the office he didn't want to think about or second-guess his wife's preferences. Tension grew between them until they seldom spoke. They stopped going out alone together. Their intimate life ended.[22]

In the story of the Smiths, the threat to practical identities posed by inadequate material support is plain. And, although no one in particular is identified as propagandizing for a narrative of (female) caregiver self-abnegation, it is clear that the Smiths have imbibed a toxic dose of the culture's general stories about who draws the lot for caregiving. It's Theresa who cuts back on her job, Robert who seems to think that he's effectively released from sharing her responsibilities. Even the way the story is told seems influenced by these stereotypes. We're told that "Robert received little attention from his wife," when the opposite might seem more accurate—Theresa did try to interact with Robert, but not in the way he preferred, so that he withdrew his attention. The Smiths' spousal identities, as well as Theresa's work-related identity, eroded. Nor is the evidence here solely narrative; studies with more general scope point in the same direction. Social scientists studying "the caregiving career" have noted that caregiving not only exerts significant pressure on the array of identities that family members maintain, but does so in a dynamic, relentlessly expanding fashion. In their study, *Profiles in Caregiving: The Unexpected Career*, Aneshensel, Zarit, and Whitlach note that "[typically] the caregiver role keeps expanding in its demands so that even with adjustments in other areas, it keeps a steady pressure on the boundaries of other roles in the constellation."[23] Thus, even creative accommodation to new demands can't ensure that the integrity of a family caregiver's other practical identities is preserved.

At the same time, the stories of the Smiths and the Levines also suggest that families regard the immense burden of intense, prolonged, and exacting care as worth bearing. This willingness can also be understood as a testimony to the importance people place on the maintenance of practical identities. For if home-based care can erode and transmute family relationships, causing, for example, distinctively spousal identities to fail, alternative institutional care carries dangers of its own. It seems fair—indeed, important—to ask whether the Smiths would have been likely to hang onto any remnant of their identities as parents if their daughter had been institutionalized.

IS THERE A RIGHT TO "FAMILY CARE"?

I've tried to show various dimensions of harm that intensive and prolonged health care provision can pose to families, while acknowledging that such care can have value to families as well. Yet the kinds of
goods that many families find in providing care to ill or disabled relatives, along with at least some of the social savings to be had from
their involvement, do not require that lives and identities be as deeply
harmed as in the stories retold and studies related here.[24] More generous, and generously available benefits, allowing family care providers
respite from their tasks would help; greater acknowledgment on the
part of the health care professions and society of the important and
expanding role of family in health care would, too. The demand that
families "spend down" to the poverty level to qualify for Medicaid
long-term care benefits seems a Draconian measure in an affluent society; need, rather than penury, could be the chief eligibility criterion.
Family leave provisions, such as those guaranteed by the Family and
Medical Leave Act, could be extended and strengthened; those who
must relinquish or cut down on paid employment for caretaking purposes could be extended taxation and retirement fund support to ease
the fiscal costs of substituting one sort of socially significant work for
another. Home-based care providers need information and a sense of
connection and appreciation; the Internet might help with these things
(assuming caregivers have sufficient time and energy to take advantage of it), and access might be subsidized for those family care providers not now on-line. If telemedicine can add to the momentum
behind refiguring the health care roles of family members, telecom-
muting might allow more family members to express their practical
identities as workers, and enjoy the stress-reducing benefits that out-
of-the-home work apparently can afford.[25]

Most of these proposals most directly target "material" conditions
of the sort that imperiled some of the Smiths' practical identities; others speak to the "expressive" conditions that damaged Carol Levine,
the withdrawal of the community uptake that diluted her social standing as a wife. Changing the social perception of family caregivers is
likely to require also changing their material conditions. If greater economic support for family caregivers made it easier for them to continue to lead rich and varied lives, it would be harder to figure them as
simply and solely the performers of those "unrelieved nasty chores."

Yet life is full of misfortunes, and not all misfortunes involve questions of justice and injustice. Many of the proposals canvassed above

could reduce the savings drawn from increased reliance on family caregiving, and tempering health care spending is a significant matter, particularly as the health care inflation engine shifts back into high gear.[26] What is it about those misfortunes faced by family members in providing health care to their relatives that distinguishes them from, say, finding oneself locked into a tedious job due to an inability to get health insurance elsewhere? Practical identities can be constrained or withheld if your salary is too small to satisfy your deep interest in contemporary art, or if your vertical leap is too short to play in the National Basketball Association, or to dance with the American Ballet Theater.

One conditional line of argument that family caregiving should be subvened by social resources is suggested by what seems a ready analogy between caregiving and illness. It is relatively commonplace among bioethicists—and apparently, among most of the people of the developed world outside the U.S.—to think that health care ranks among the most important human needs, more akin to the need for education than to a hankering for collecting period instruments or going on ski vacations. Maintaining my health, curing my illnesses, repairing my dysfunctions, easing my pain, staving off my mortality— all these tasks are caught up with a class of possible misfortunes that it is seemingly appropriate to provide for out of a community's joint resources; health, or at least access to the health care system, is a kind of good that a just society will make available to all its members.

Among the needs that people face, why is health care reasonably thought to enjoy this special status? One popular argument is that health care aims at securing a primary good—a good that aids us in the pursuit of every more specific vision of the good. I may, for example, pin my hopes for a good life on acquiring a gracious home, a prestigious job, and a charming and compliant spouse; you may regard all this as so much fluff, as a frivolous or even as an immoral set of goals for a human life, preferring to build communities of resistance to entrenched powers and practices, to undermine patriarchal and capitalist systems. But we will both do better in achieving our aims if we are healthy, and we both have a better chance of being healthy if we have reliable access to health care resources. A society professedly neutral among its members' conceptions of the good might justify insuring access to health care by trading on the "plasticity" of the benefit of health.

A related, although distinguishable idea—the notion that health care is key to the maintenance of a "normal opportunity range"—has been prominently advocated by Norman Daniels.[27] Noting that some (a rare

few, presumably) may hold conceptions of the good that are not abet-
ted by health, he argues that the ability to change your plan of life
within a range normal for your species and to which you are otherwise
suited, is also rationally regarded as a significant good. If anyone were
indifferent to it, that would presumably be because she either had no
interest in how she lived at all, or because she was absolutely convinced that her present plan of life was in no need of assessment or
improvement. Holding appropriate allocation of social resources hos-
tage to nihilism seems too strong a requirement, and it is unlikely that
assumptions of infallibility are consistent with practical rationality. If
the ability to revise your plan of life is an especially significant good,
then interventions designed to maintain or restore normal species
function—that is, health care—may well be required for you to have
that kind of opportunity. Neither notional nor practical revision may
be possible if you're seriously ill.

The analogous argument for socially supporting family health care
provision hinges on the view that the ability to form and to maintain a
practical identity is as likely to be a primary good as is health. There
are close ties between the idea of practical identity and the notion of a
normal opportunity range. Illnesses and traumas are not the only
impairments in our normal species function that can block our revising
(or living out) a conception of the good. Forming practical identities
is part of what is normal to our species, and the ability to do it is intimately caught up with our opportunity range.

Indeed, the collection of practical identities open to a person might
be seen as a way of specifying the "range of opportunity normal to
our species and to which [that] individual is otherwise suited." While
some practical identities will be less significant to a person than others, the same could be said about the impairments caused by different
illnesses. Accordingly, what undermines a person's ability to form or
maintain central practical identities is therefore, in general terms, as
morally significant as what threatens her health. If the appeal to primary goods or normal opportunity ranges makes the provision of
health care a matter of justice, then, by parity of argument, it would
motivate a similar conclusion with respect to provision of support for
family-based care providers, at least in a society whose health care
system relies on exacting forms of family-provided care.

It might be argued that, whereas a person cannot simply walk away
from her ill body, she can refuse family caregiving responsibilities and
their potential risks to practical identities. But this both understates our
freedom with respect to ourselves, and overstates our freedom with

respect to our families. Failure to provide care needed by a family member may be, for many, just as destructive of central practical identities as taking a lethal overdose.

I conclude that if arguments based on such notions as "primary goods" or "normal opportunity ranges" are successful in showing that access to a reasonable level of health care is guaranteed by an appropriate understanding of distributive justice, then access to a reasonable level of support for families providing burdensome health care is equally strongly supported. In the U.S., of course, such arguments have not been effective politically, regardless of their philosophical merits.

But the conditional argument sketched here is also more ambitious than strictly required to show that "drafting" families to replace health care professionals is unjust. Considerations of ambiguous agency notwithstanding, the strategy of greatly increased reliance on family-based care that constricts opportunities to form, revise, and live out practical identities is scarcely the result of natural causes. Rather, it results from a collection of decisions to shift costs from government or private insurers to families, a cheap and readily available labor source. That some family members may see themselves as having a moral obligation to take on these jobs does not imply that the social arrangements that put them in such positions are acceptable.

There are, as I have tried to show, serious considerations justifying socially funded efforts to ease the burdens on family caregivers quite apart from arguments that rely on how prone families are to exploitation. However, the fact that the particular situation facing U.S. families now is a result of the efforts of morally responsible agents—insurers, employers, employees—trying to make their own lot easier needs a positive moral justification that has not been forthcoming. Pleading ignorance about the impact of these decisions is increasingly implausible. At least when prolonged and intense family care provision is at issue, then, reasonably affluent societies have as stringent a duty to provide families with the kind of support that will allow caregivers to maintain central practical identities, as they do to provide basic health care. Further, if people in the U.S. benefit by the kind of care increasingly loaded on to family members—and even in the absence of a nationally insured system of universally accessible health care, it seems that we do—then we have a justice-based reason to keep the provision of that care from being gravely harmful to features of human life that are very widely, and very deeply, valued.

Sadly, appeals to justice sometimes lack pragmatic clout. Yet, where justice flags, prudence sometimes prevails. Finding yourself called upon to provide prolonged, difficult health care to those you love is not a remote possibility. Very many people have very good reasons to take steps to better the odds that our identities will remain rich and varied, that our lives as caregivers will not need to be lives of heroic sacrifice.

NOTES

1. See Katharine Levit, Cathy Cowan, Helen Lazenby, Arthur Sensenig, Patricia McDonnell, Jean Stiller, and Anne Martin, "Health Spending in 1998: Signals of Change," *Health Affairs* 19, no. 1 (2000): 124–32; and Milt Freudenham, "HMO Costs Spur Employers to Shift Plans," *New York Times*, 6 September 2000, 1(A).

2. Carol Levine, "Home Sweet Hospital: The Nature and Limits of Private Responsibilities for Home Health Care," *Journal of Aging and Health Care* 11 (1999): 341–59.

3. See the papers in *Bringing the Hospital Home: Ethical and Social Implications of High-Tech Home; Care*, ed. John Arras (Baltimore, Md.: Johns Hopkins University Press, 1995), and Keith A. Bauer, "Home-based Telemedicine: A Survey of Ethical Issues," *Cambridge Quarterly of Health Care Ethics* 10, no. 2 (April 2001): 137–46.

4. Levine, "Home Sweet Hospital," 342.

5. John Rawls, *A Theory of Justice* (Cambridge, Mass.: Harvard University Press, 1971), 27.

6. Rawls, *A Theory of Justice*, 3.

7. See Salvator Minuchin, *Families; and Family Therapy* (Cambridge, Mass.: Harvard University Press, 1974), and Hilde Lindemann Nelson and James Lindemann Nelson, *The Patient in the Family* (New York: Routledge, 1995).

8. Some theorists of the family are quite convinced, however, that there are no good moral reasons for families not to become more formal, their interchanges governed by contract rather than implicit patterns of understanding and practice. See, for instance, Susan Okin, *Justice, Gender and the Family* (New York: Basic Books, 1989).

9. What constitutes "one family" is itself also open to debate. Late-appearing "long-lost relatives" who assert authority over health care decisions, and homosexual or otherwise queer partners, are just two fairly prominent instances where who is "really family" is sometimes disputed.

10. Diemut Bubeck argues to this effect in her *Care, Gender and Justice* (Oxford: Clarendon Press, 1995), 171–85.

11. Christine Korsgaard, *The Sources of Normativity* (Cambridge: Cambridge University Press, 1996), 101.

12. Korsgaard, *Sources*, 101.

13. Brody, 1990.

14. More direct discussions of gender justice in families can be found in Okin, *Justice, Gender and the Family*; and Nelson and Nelson, *The Patient in the Family*; a good recent discussion is Eva Feder Kittay, *Love's Labor* (New York: Routledge, 1999). For an extended discussion of the relationships among identity, agency, and justice, see Hilde Lindemann Nelson, *Damaged Identities, Narrative Repair* (Ithaca, N.Y.: Cornell University Press, 2001).

15. Carol Levine, "The Loneliness of the Long-Term Care Giver," *New England Journal of Medicine* 340 (1999): 1587–90.

16. Levine, "Long-Term Care Giver," 1587.

17. Levine, "Long-Term Care Giver," 1588.

18. Carol Levine, "Night Shift," *Ms.* 10 (2000), 44.

19. Levine, "Night Shift," 44.

20. My analysis here is much influenced by Hilde Lindemann Nelson, *Damaged Identities, Narrative Repair*.

21. Carol Levine, *Rough Crossings: Family Caregivers' Odysseys through the Health Care System* (New York: United Hospital Fund, 1998). The literature on family caregiving and dementia is also full of similar stories. For representative examples, showing families seeking ways to both care for relatives and to preserve other significant features of their lives, see James Lindemann Nelson and Hilde Lindemann Nelson, *Alzheimer's: Answers to Hard Questions for Families* (New York: Doubleday, 1996).

22. Levine, *Rough Crossings*, 24.

23. Carol Aneshensel, Steven Zarit, and Carol Whitlach, *Profiles in Caregiving: The Unexpected Career* (San Diego, Calif.: Academic Press, 1995).

24. A fuller story of the impact on families and on practical identities of intensive tending of ill relatives would require the input of those who have studied family caretaking for disabled children, and of those family members themselves. Some have maintained that families involved in this type of caregiving do not fare notably worse than families otherwise engaged. See, for instance, Philip Ferguson, Alan Gartner, Dorothy Lipsky, "The Experience of Disability in Families: A Synthesis of Research and Parent Narratives," in *Prenatal Genetic Testing and Disability Rights*, ed. Erik Parens and Adrienne Asch (Washington, D.C.: Georgetown University Press, 2000), 72–94.

25. See Levine, "Night Shift," 45.

26. David Rosenbaum, "What if There is No Cure for Health Care's Ills?" *New York Times*, 10 September 2000, section 4, 1.

27. Norman Daniels, *Just Health Care* (Cambridge: Cambridge University Press, 1985).

4

Death's Gender

Death, Wallace Stevens tells us in "Sunday Morning," is the "mother of beauty."[1] For David Jones, death is a prostitute; his World War I epic poem, *In Parenthesis*, speaks of "sweet sister death" who strides about the battlefield with "strumpet confidence."[2] And Diana Tietjens Meyers tells us that art portrays the face of death as the face of an old woman, the face of an old woman as the face of death.[3]

SEXING DEATH

These invocations of poetry and the graphic arts suggest one sense in which death has a gender: death, like nature, chaos, the body, emotion, and evil, has been connected in cultural imaginaries with the female.[4] Any strict identification of this kind might be contested; of course there seems nothing so very feminine about the Grim Reaper, for example, and Milton made Death the son of Sin by her father Satan. My purpose here, though, is not to sort out the various gendered forms in which the idea of death has been cloaked. I will be interested in a different sense in which death might be gendered—in whether the gender of those who die might not alter the character of death.

This might seem an odd enterprise. Death could well strike us, as it apparently did Epicurus and Lucretius, as preeminently characterless. Or, if it has anything in the way of a character—if it is best understood, say, as a total and permanent privation of all that could possibly matter to a person—that character would seem uniform, and uniformly nega-

71

tive. Although timing and circumstances of dying alter radically from person to person, everyone dies alike, and, so far as can be determined in the order of nature, all the dead fare the same: a dead person has no further experiences of any kind; a dead body decays. Neither gender nor any other distinguishing feature of people would seem to affect this one whit.

Odd though it may seem, this is precisely the enterprise I want to take on here. Much of what I will attempt involves showing that death is diverse in ways that the leading philosophical accounts do not fully accommodate. I begin by showing how inviting it is for philosophers who are interested in the moral relationships among different age groups or differently aged people to make both too much and not enough of mortality. These analyses have special, and sometimes worrisome, implications for women, but my particular interest here will be in showing how these thinkers more or less explicitly rely on inadequate understandings of how death constitutes a harm to persons.

I then explore how gender may in fact be relevant to what kind of harms death constitutes to us mortals. Here, I will be drawing on the idea that systematic differences in what people value are relevant to the magnitude of death's harm, and as well on the idea that gender differences may track those systematic value differences more or less closely.

Finally, I want at least to rough out the outlines of three implications of the account developed here. One concerns a characteristic move in well-known theoretical efforts to use age as a device for making distributive justice decisions. The other two concern practice: little-noted gender biases in some of the most prominent cultural strategies for finding consolation in the face of mortality, and equally obscure dangers in the shifts in values that may accompany ways many women live today.

DEATH, AGE, CLASS

The literary critic Morris Zapp, one of the characters in David Lodge's series of academic novels, finds that he has rather lost his enthusiasm for poststructuralism after being kidnapped by terrorists. Zapp explains this by saying that his abduction has taught him a lesson: "Death is the one concept you can't deconstruct."[5] A number of contemporary philosophers seem to agree with Zapp's idea that death is "on the other side of language." At least, their accounts of death and its significance seem to deny to death the multiplicity that has recently been recognized as a signal feature of other socially, politically, and morally important concepts. For example, unlike, "race" or "gender," "death" is not often portrayed as something differently shaped for different people by different collusions of social powers, values, and practices.

Age As Superfact

Daniel Callahan, for example, who has written with considerable sensitivity about the way in which social circumstances and shared meanings might render dying "wild," "tame," or "peaceful,"[6] develops his account of what the old and young owe each other in a way that makes the issue of the proximity to death the single most important feature that both defines what it is to be old and gives the old their characteristic moral tasks. Dying may be a complex and socially mediated phenomenon, but death itself is simpler; as a general matter, its significance for Callahan is crucially conditioned by age. The death of the young is typically "tragic"; the death of the old, "tolerable." The old have already enjoyed the opportunities to discharge their duties and to gain the goods life provides; if, sadly, their personal or social circumstances have made it impossible for them to do so, this situation is not likely to be remedied simply by living longer.[7]

Frances Kamm, in trying to determine how justly to adjudicate contests over scarce, life-prolonging resources, makes how long one has already lived a crucial criterion for determining the gravity of one's need to go on living: the longer the life, the less need for more. For when it comes to the allocation of life-prolonging resources, the younger, solely because they are younger, are generally the "worse off" when compared to anyone at all older.[8] And Norman Daniels, who sets himself the task of justifying systems of health care allocation that favor the young over the old as age groups, notes that all of us who do not die prematurely move through all life's stages. He argues that therefore we can sensibly imagine distributing a fixed set of resources throughout the different periods of our lives. From that perspective, he maintains, it would be irrational to prefer an allocation of social resources designed to extend our lives when already old to an allocation designed to improve the chances that we will get to be old in the first place.[9] Again, this assumes that death's significance is, in the general case, a function of age alone. It is worth more to forestall death at an early age than to stave off a later death.

It has hardly been lost on feminists that basing social duties and notions of justice on age (in Daniels and Callahan, specifically on being elderly) affects women in particular, as women have a greater chance than men of becoming old, of being old for a long time, and of requiring a good deal of health care during their lives as elderly people. That women's stake in these theories is persistently undertheonzed by their authors has been argued repeatedly in the literature.[10] What I want to feature here, however, is that, despite their differences, all of these writers regard death as "aged"—that is, the kind of harm death is to a person, or the seriousness of one's claims to the resources required to avoid it, is dominantly affected by age. For none of them is it otherwise marked—not by ethnicity, not by class, and not by gender.

The theoretical attraction of the idea that one's age is so strongly relevant to the allocation of social resources is clearly enormous. If one is in the business of trying to figure out how to divide limited resources justly, and there is a "superfact" to save the day, so very much the better. By "superfact" I mean a fact that characterizes a set of people in a manner so relevant to distribution of goods or assignment of duties that none of their other traits, nor any of the traits of potential claimants not in that group can, singly or in combination, defeat its dispositive relevance. Who in the distributive justice game wouldn't be intrigued at the prospect of such a device?

Suppose, however, that the general respects in which death is a harm are not uniform, but vary according to considerations other than age. If such were the case, it would be arbitrary to give to age superfact status. Michael Neill's book *Issues of Death* suggests that death's harms may indeed vary along other dimensions. In trying to make better sense of English Renaissance tragedy, Neill argues that one of the most unsettling features about death to Renaissance Europeans was its rough egalitarianism; aristocrat and pauper died and decomposed alike.[11] This was taken to be unnatural, an outrageous cancellation of fundamental structures of meaning. Neill quotes John Donne to good effect in making this point:

[W]e must all pass this posthume death, this death after death, nay this death after burial, this dissolution after dissolution, this death of corruption and putrefaction, of vermiculation and incineration, of dissolution and dispersion in and from the grave, when those bodies that have been the children of royal parents and the parents of royal children, must say with Job, *to corruption, thou art my father,* and *to the worm, thou art my mother and my sister.* Miserable riddle, when the same worm must be my mother, my sister and my self! Miserable incest, when I must be married to my mother and my sister, and be both father and mother to my own mother and sister, beget and bear that worm which is all that miserable penury; when my mouth shall be filled with dust, and the worm shall feed, and feed sweetly, upon me; when the ambitious man shall have no satisfaction, if the poorest alive tread upon him, nor the poorest receive any contentment in being made equal to princes, for they shall be equal but in dust. . . . This is the most inglorious and contemptible vilification, the most deadly and preemptory nullification of man that we can consider.[12]

This is, to say no more, a complex piece of prose, not least in its use of gendered images. But Neill sees Donne's main theme to be repugnance at death's role as the Great Leveler. His historical work suggests two points. One is that *widely spread social understandings can contribute to the ways in which death is taken to be a harm.* While our own contemporaries are not free of the temptation to see structures of social privilege as reflections of the natural order, I suspect that death's being a common fate is less annoying to people today than some of its other features. This is surely not because we are nowadays indifferent about our place in hierarchies. Perhaps it indicates that we have become more instrumental about them than were many among our cultural predecessors. Being above others is widely prized, but largely to the extent that it secures one greater access to other things that are coveted: income, power, prestige, and the rest of the litany. Death either eliminates these goods or is irrelevant to them, and it's the absence of the goods that is taken to be important nowadays. That death also eliminates hierarchical patterns of distribution of such goods is, for many of us, largely beside the point. Insofar as there is a shift in the reasons why hierarchical orders are valued, the response to their loss may shift as well.

The second point that seems implicit in Neill is that *people's place in a social structure can also affect the ways in which death is taken to harm them.* Donne suggests that the poor have no consolation in becoming no worse dust than their betters in life, but I cannot help but think that death's egalitarianism was at least somewhat more nettlesome to those who would be going down in the (under)world than to those for whom death was a form, however limited, of upward mobility—death's "preemptory nullification" is more of a problem, that is, for princes than for paupers.

However it stood with people in Renaissance Europe, Neill's historical work allows us to imagine a way in which social understandings
and specifically class position might well affect the respects in which
people saw death as a harm. It thereby prepares the ground for a view
of death's harms more complex than that envisaged by Callahan,
Kamm, or Daniels, one that acknowledges the relevance of social
markers. If death, or at least its harms, can be class-sensitive in
Renaissance England, why not gender-sensitive now?

Death's Sting

Old aristocrats in Renaissance Europe no doubt had better access to
whatever life-prolonging technologies were then on offer than did
young paupers; could they have justified their advantage with the
claim that, due to their class position, death constituted a greater harm
to them than to the youthful poor?

This may strike us inheritors of the Enlightenment as counterintuitive, and there is a natural way of accounting for that response. It
might be that different groups of people *have feared* death for different
reasons, but it does not follow that these social beliefs about death
reflect differences in what *actually* makes death a harm. Nor is it clear
what the ethical implications of mere beliefs about death's harmfulness might be. The real problem, it might seem, is to show whether
death itself is a harm of a different kind to some people than to others.

The Goods of Experience and Action

There is, of course, an old and surprisingly tough question about
whether, and if so in what respects, it is a bad thing to die at all. This
question is seldom discussed—at least nowadays—in ways that would
suggest that death might be a different thing for people differently situated and constituted.[13] While I have drawn from Neill's work the suggestion that class location might change at least some of the respects
in which death is harmful, I imagine this idea would not be well
received by those philosophers who have done the most conspicuous
and explicit recent work on how death might be a harm: I have in mind
particularly Thomas Nagel, whose article "Death" is surely something
of a contemporary classic on this question,[14] and Kamm, who has
thought through this question very thoroughly indeed.[15] Both would
likely distinguish between, on the one hand, the varieties of disturbing
beliefs that may be associated with death—that is, that death removes

essential distinctions, or, to take a more familiar example, the fear of eternal damnation—and, on the other, those considerations in which the harmfulness of death really resides, quite apart from what anyone believes—that is, because it forever deprives us of all possibility of the goods of experience and action, to use Kamm's formulation. What makes death bad in fact and not fancy, as Nagel and Kamm see it, is the same for all of us.

But *was* the Renaissance belief that death cancels out important distinctions simply false, and is the view of Nagel, as amended by Kamm, that death deprives us of the goods of experience and action (and makes things "all over" for us) in contrast straightforwardly true? So far as can be known, *both* the Renaissance and the Nagel-Kamm characterizations are correct—if there is a difference, it is that people care much less about death as a leveler than they do about death as, so to speak, an extinguisher. Different facts about death affect different people at different times in different ways, it seems, and the moral is that we need a less generic account of why death is so nasty than either Nagel or even Kamm provides.

Kamm's own formulation of what death takes from us provides a glimpse of what that alternative might be like. She highlights the point that death takes away a particular kind of goods—not "all possible goods," but the "goods of experience and action."[16] This distinction itself suggests the possibility that the severity of death's sting might vary as a function of the extent to which one valued the goods of experience and action vis-à-vis unexperienced goods. Kamm develops a variant on this theme; she notes that the "true goods" of wisdom and good character, while they make life better, are "to a large degree complete in themselves once one has them," and says that they are best regarded as ways of being rather than as ways of acting or experiencing.[17] Such goods, which are among the most important things in life, are the least threatened by death.

Goods Outside Awareness and Action

But these Socratic virtues are not the only things that may have value independently of experience and action. There are, for example, possible states of affairs that neither affect nor are affected by particular people, yet about which people are far from indifferent. I, for example, would much rather it be the case that the future fifty generations hence include the existence and flourishing of many human beings living in harmony with each other, other animals, and their environment, than have the future be depleted of all that gives the present grace. I would rather it not be the case that I am at this moment being viciously slandered, even to people who don't believe a word of it, and even if I should never find out about the matter.

At first blush, some philosophers might not accept these examples as pointing to goods of unawareness and inaction. Both examples are introduced with a phrase that seems to relate a state of affairs to my wants. But what I intend to convey with these examples is that I judge a future state of the world in which justice flourishes and the lion lies down with the lamb and suchlike, to be better than less pacific and equitable alternatives—not, ex hypothesis, better for me, but better for those who inhabit that world, or, perhaps, better objectively. I think of a state of the world that includes my being selected as a target for foul yet-forever-undetected-by-me calumny to be worse perhaps for those who have to hear such drivel, or for those who spout it, or perhaps just worse simpliciter, than a similar state of the world that contains instead someone holding me up to the sort of criticism I deserve.

While sentiments of this sort are fairly widespread, it is quite possible that people might place more or less store in values not involving action or experience. It's not hard to imagine someone—call him Jack—quite willing to say that he was not indifferent to the state of the world fifty generations hence, but all of whose true enthusiasms revolve around what he experienced and what he did. I think it also possible to imagine someone much more engaged by unexperienced goods—call her Jill. For Jill, her children's flourishing is enormously valuable. While she enjoys watching them at it, fundamentally, it doesn't much matter to her at what time their lives are going well—now, or twenty years after her death. Jill might well prefer an arrangement in which the children's lives go somewhat less well during her own life, if that were necessary for matters to turn out very much better for them after her death.

Noting that the inevitability of a catastrophe does not necessarily make it any the less bad, Nagel famously concludes "Death" with the phrase, "It may be that a bad end is in store for all of us." After all, death is an "abrupt cancellation of indefinitely extensive possible goods."[18] Nagel may have Jack's number—he may indeed be cruising toward a bad end. Jill's prospects, however, may not be quite so dire. Not all of what matters deeply to her is quite so vulnerable to death's privations. Even the permanent loss of what are in principle indefinitely extendable goods does not necessarily leave one in a bad state. Much depends upon what is retained and how it is valued. Of course,

Jill's special engagement with unexperienced goods leaves open the possibility that she is liable to harms related to her death of a kind against which Jack is better armored—suppose, for example, that her children's lives go on the whole badly after her death. But at least with respect to the currently leading philosophical accounts of the matter, Jill seems the better off.

I further want to suggest that the reasons why Jack runs into this problem and Jill does not are not completely idiosyncratic. There are social forces that incline Jack and Jill to value as they do—forces that are not accidentally related to their genders.

HOW WE DIE: CAREER SELVES AND SERIATIM SELVES

In Harold Pinter's *Moonlight,* the dying Andy lies in his bed among the shards of his life. Estranged from his sons, disconnected from his friends, he and his wife exchange bitter boasts about their infidelities. All he has to cling to is the most important feature of what he has been:

> I sweated over a hot desk all the working life and nobody ever found a flaw in my working procedures. Nobody uncovered the slightest hint of negligence or misdemeanor. Never. . . . *I* was a first class civil servant. I was admired and respected. I do not say I was loved. I didn't want to be loved. Love is an attribute no civil servant worth his salt would give house room to. It's redundant. An excrescence. No, no, *I'll* tell you what *I* was. *I* was an envied and feared force in the temples of the just.[19]

In Margaret Walker's *Moral Understandings*, Andy—or, rather, his ghost—makes another appearance, albeit anonymously.[20] Walker discusses the prevalence within moral theory of a particular kind of self disturbingly like Andy, which she styles the "career self." Roughly sketched, a career self sees his life (aspirationally, in any event) as a unified field, in which particular enterprises, values, and relationships are (in principle) coordinated in the form of a "rational life plan" (à la Rawls), or a "quest" (to use the term favored by Alastair MacIntyre and Charles Taylor), or a "project" (as Bernard Williams is wont to say). It's tempting to describe such lives in terms of the chapter titles of a conventionally structured novel: "The Years of Preparation," followed by "The Years of Struggle" and "The Years of Achievement," and finally, as the telltale compression of the pages warn us, "The

Years of Retirement." There is a shape to this life, both in principle and in practice: you go up through the ranks, get tenure, make professor, and then get an endowed chair; you finish law school, get a good clerkship, become an associate at a top firm, and then make partner; an MBA, a key to the executive washroom, the million-dollar circle. Such conceptions of life typically put great stress on agency and individuality (I exercise *my* agency to envisage and attain my goals, slaying such dragons as have the temerity to present themselves along the way), on what I experience myself as getting, keeping, and doing, as well as on relatively distinct tasks for distinct phases of life.

THE GOODS OF AGENCY VERSUS
THE GOODS OF RELATIONSHIP

Now, if this is at all on target, it would be natural to regard the loss of the goods of individual agency and experience as heavy indeed for career selves—something akin, perhaps, to the impact of the leveling effect of death on Renaissance aristocrats. It would also seem natural to see old age as having something of a unified and distinct character. Typically, it will be the time after the dragons have been slain and the quest fulfilled, and the task remaining is to make a graceful exit. Thus, the career self trope fits nicely with Callahan's general analysis of age as a unified category robust enough to support a distinct set of duties. It also coheres with Nagel's and Kamm's discussion of the harm of death, further supporting Walker's point that the career self notion is theoretically ubiquitous, haunting the thought of otherwise very different philosophers. But a good part of Walker's point in introducing the career self notion, and drawing attention to its largely unmotivated presence at the heart of the thought of writers otherwise maintaining importantly different commitments, is to point out the possibility of living a life in ways importantly different from that described with notions such as "career," "quest," "project," or "plan"—indeed, of pointing out that such lives are in fact lived.

Hilde Lindemann Nelson has in discussion used the phrase "living life seriatim" to designate an alternative to the career trajectory. I take her to mean seeing life less as an overall unified project and more as a set of fits and starts. For "seriatim selves," what death portends by way of harms, and the idea of the appropriate tasks of later life as well, might be different from what they are for career selves. The career self's big job is over as he enters his twilight years, and the final task is to fill out the remains of the day with some dignity. But the seriatim self may see her life as made up of many jobs, lots of them quite big enough, thank you, but none necessarily life-defining, nor especially valued for the particular role they play in contributing to the achievement of a "rational plan" for the whole.

Rather, there's the time of going to school, and then the time of getting married and dealing with pregnancies and children. After that, there may be a time of going back to school, a time of having a job apart from family obligations. But that may not last, because there may be a time of changing locations because of the more exigent career demands of a spouse who is a career self. There may then be a time of starting out doing something else, and a time of caring for one's parents, and perhaps of tending the grandchildren.

The connections between being a career or a seriatim self and how one values the goods of experience and agency vis-à-vis the non-exponential dimensions of the goods of relationship are, of course, not logically necessary. A career self could certainly pursue a seamless project of exemplary selflessness, in which expressing one's own agency and having gratifying experiences were largely incidental, not to the main point at all. A seriatim self could find goods of action and experience the most fulfilling feature of every stop along her variegated way. Yet, as Cheshire Calhoun has pointed out, nonlogical connections can be as philosophically important as logically necessary ones.[21] The patterns of social practice and understandings that make career selves so prevalent, in both theory and practice, are part of what she might call an "ideology of the moral life" that installs the view that there is nothing so natural (at least for those paradigmatic moral agents, otherwise privileged men) as striving to impose one's own vision on life, and that many of the relationships that come our way will be with people with similar desires, leading to something of a premium on cultivating what Aristotle called "friends for use."

Agency and experience are big themes all the way through the pertinent philosophical accounts; there is surely nothing contemplative in the connotation of "quest" or even in the less dramatic "project" or "rational life plan." They are big themes as well in the real lives that both give rise to and approximate these idealizations. But a seriatim self has escaped, more or less, the ideological pressures, as well as the ideological and material rewards that encourage people to identify themselves with their careers, and hence may live a life both more shaped by contingencies than by the expression of personal agency and more involved in relationships prized intrinsically, not because of their role in the agent's achieving her quest. Individual experience and agency are surely important to pursuing and nurturing relationships, but they may not be as important as the site where the value of such pursuits reside. Seriatim selves may, then, place a greater importance on the goods of relationship, rather than the goods of agency and experience.

I don't mean to deny that creating, preserving, and getting the good out of relationships won't importantly involve what people do, think, and feel. Nor that the social forces that have inclined more women than men to lives oriented relationally and lived seriatim are benign in intent or effect; quite the contrary. But lives so lived may have a special access to the values of relationship, and among the goods of those relationships that are not altogether a matter of who is useful to whom, one must surely be an appreciation of the significance of the other quite on her own terms, not as a function of what makes me happy.[22] People who manage to make the good of others central to their lives in this way are importantly invested in something robust enough to withstand their deaths.

DEATH AND WOMEN'S AGING WITH DIGNITY

Morris Zapp was wrong. Death doesn't wear its meaning on its face univocal, stable, and uncontestable. Nor is age the only dimension along which its significance varies. There is reason to believe that its character is altered according to one's position in the system of class differences, and reason, too, to think that it alters with one's position in the system of gender differences, or at least that gender closely tracks patterns of human valuing with which the significance of death more directly varies.

I have already suggested that very influential age-based theories of distributive justice make the mistake of supposing that the harmfulness of death varies as a general matter with age alone, but I've yet to draw out the implications of the error, particularly as they affect women who are old. I have also implied that ignoring the sense in which death is gendered has unfortunate implications for social practices that involve women distinctively; something more needs to be said about that, as well.

Aging, Dignity, and Justice

Most feminist assessments of theories of intergenerational justice have been concerned that the interests of aging women were particularly at risk. In suggesting that at least many women may not be as vulnerable to losing the goods of action and experience as are many men, this feminist concern seems to have been given a curious twist.

In my view, however, the real lesson here is that handing out resources in ways that favor the young cannot be justified as straightforwardly as proponents would intend. If old people tend to differ by gender in the ways in which they are threatened by death, it does not follow that we should simply accept the framework of age rationing and deduct further "points" for being female as well as elderly. Such a framework rests on the misleading idea that the moral significance of selected human traits, such as age or gender, can be measured in a common scale, in a way largely detached from the full moral complexity of human life. This analytic structure needs to be questioned more rigorously. In figuring out how to direct health care budgets or hand out transplantable livers, comparing the stringency of the claims of the young qua young to those of the old qua old is a form of "false totalization," and thus is disrespectful, particularly (though not solely) to people who happen to be old. Avoiding such disrespect does not require abandoning the notion that age is relevant to issues of how to allocate scarce goods fairly; but to make age determinative is not only disrespectful, it is distracting. Making age a superfact oversimplifies the task of achieving justice in the distribution of scarce goods, but that's not the whole of the problem. So understood, the focus on age obscures other issues that are at least equally important. Why are we finding ourselves playing off Medicaid (medical support for children and the indigent) against Medicare (medical support for the elderly) in the first place? Why does health care cost as much as it does? Why do we so obsess about medicine, when the aggregate well-being may be more reliably secured by enhancing social environments? And, perhaps most radically, how would medicine and its social setting look if the central role of the goods of experience and agency in many people's lives were challenged, and hence the harm of death—or, at least the harm most theoretically apparent to philosophers now—diminished generally?

Gender and the Forms of Consolation

It seems reasonable to think that the forms of hope and consolation on offer in cultures would be specially tailored to the kinds of selves those cultures particularly prize. If, in the dominant culture, social power and authority are disproportionately in the hands of career selves, we might expect important strategies to include authoritative promises that what death crucially removes will yet be restored; that there is agency and experience beyond the grave.

This, of course, is just what we do find. Stories of personal survival, beatific visions, and resurrections of the body are not the only ways in which cultures offer hope and solace to their participants, but they clearly have had pride of place in Western societies for many centuries.[23] As important as these stories have been, however, they do little to highlight the resilience to death's harms that tend to come with ways of valuing that put less stress on action and experience. I don't mean to suggest that only hard-driving CEOs have found notions of heaven attractive; I'd be surprised if very many people, however marked by gender or class or ethnicity or age, were altogether indifferent to the goods of action and experience, and of course, certain actions and experiences constitute an important part of the value of relationships, even if they do not exhaust that value. But a more equitable society, and in particular a society with more on offer for the variety of people who are facing death soon, would do well to fill its collective imaginary with a greater variety of ways of thinking about the end of life. People who place more store on goods whose value is not altogether a matter of whether or not they themselves have certain experiences would be better served if more public discourse about death pointed to the enduring significance of such goods, about how their goodness can be relatively independent of awareness or even of temporal location.

It would be a start if the very notion that death's harm can be, at least in part, a function of what and how a person values, were itself a more readily recognizable idea. To some extent, this was a common theme to the ancient philosophers who took philosophy's task to be therapeutic; now, we leave therapy largely to medicine, trusting it to deliver us from death. About this, Dan Callahan is absolutely right—it is not going to happen. Maybe it is time again to look to philosophy for deliverance.[24]

Gender and the Sort of Selves We Are

Above, I've entered a plea that the resources society makes available to those facing death—proximately, at least people who are old; ultimately, everyone—should be deployed in a fashion more responsive to the different ways in which death is a harm to us. In fact, it would be all to the good if more of us accepted the very possibility that something potentially a matter of human control—how and what we value—is strongly relevant to the kind of harms death presents to us. This would hold open the chance for people to shift to less classically individualist "career self" oriented patterns; if it also meant that a more egalitarian world led to more people adopting what had previously been characterized as feminine ways of living, no harm done.

Alas, what may be happening is just the reverse. If the Western world today is not more egalitarian in general, it at least presents more opportunity for women, particularly those privileged in racial, class, and other respects, to be more visible and more powerful in areas of social life from which they had previously been more rigorously restricted. This is certainly to be applauded, but everything has the defects of its qualities. It may be the case that women who today are not yet old, and perhaps therefore in a position to take greater advantage of new opportunities than their foremothers, may find themselves lacking in some of the strengths women now elderly tend to possess. In short, they may find themselves in this respect to be more like men—not necessarily in that they will die sooner than their foremothers, but that, having had as central parts of their lives the kind of careers traditional for men, they may die valuing more as men have valued. There are surely features in the lives of many women with careers that would tend to resist this assimilation. But it would be unfortunate if a more egalitarian world means a world in which more people are more like what many men traditionally have been, and in which the question of death's gender has been decisively settled.

ACKNOWLEDGMENTS

Perhaps more than is usually the case, it is important to acknowledge that no one else can be held responsible for these ideas. However, I have received an enormous amount of help from Hilde Lindemann Nelson, Margaret Walker, Ellen Robinson, and the participants in the wonderfully stimulating Conference on Ethical Issues in Women's Aging with Dignity, held at the Ethics Center, the University of South Florida, in February 1998. I must in particular mention Sara Ruddick and Diana Tietjens Meyers. William Ruddick was also kind enough to read a late draft and share his thoughtful impressions with me. I wish I could have profited more from all their good counsel. Finally, I am also much beholden to Eric Nelson's performance as Andy in a pro-

duction of Pinter's *Moonlight* performed at the College of St. Bene-
dict, St. Joseph, Minnesota, in March 1998.

NOTES

1. Wallace Stevens, "Sunday Morning," in *The Collected Poems of Wallace Stevens* (New York, Knopf, 1954), 66–70.
2. David Jones, *In Parenthesis* (New York: Chilmark, 1962), 162.
3. Diana Tietjens Meyers, *"Miroir, Memoire, Mirage*: Appearance, Aging, and Women," in *Mother Time: Ethical Issues in Women and Aging*, ed. Margaret Urban Walker (Lanham, Md.: Rowman & Littlefield, 1999). See also chapter 6 of Meyers, *Gender in the Mirror: Cultural Imagery & Women's Agency* (Oxford: Oxford University Press, 2002).
4. For discussion of this theme, see Genevieve Lloyd, *The Man of Reason: "Male" and "Female" in Western Philosophy* (Minneapolis: University of Minnesota Press, 1984).
5. David Lodge, *Small World* (New York: Warner Books, 1984), 373.
6. Daniel Callahan, *The Troubled Dream of Life* (New York: Simon & Schuster, 1993).
7. Daniel Callahan, *Setting Limits* (New York: Simon & Schuster, 1987). His characterization of a tolerable death is given on p. 66.
8. Frances M. Kamm, *Morality, Mortality, vol. 1: Death and Whom to Save from It* (New York: Oxford University Press, 1993).
9. Norman Daniels, *Am I My Parent's Keeper?* (New York: Oxford University Press, 1988). See also "The Prudential Life-Span Account of Justice Across Generations," in his *Justice and Justification: Reflective Equilibrium in Theory and Practice* (Cambridge: Cambridge University Press, 1996), 257–83.
10. For feminist discussion of Callahan, see Nora Kizer Bell, "If Age Becomes a Standard for Rationing Health Care . . ." in *Feminist Perspectives in Medical Ethics*, ed. Helen Bequaert Holmes and Laura Purdy (Bloomington: Indiana University Press, 1992), 82–90; Kathleen M. Dixon, "Oppressive Limits: Callahan's Foundation Myth," *Journal of Medicine and Philosophy* 19, no. 6 (1994): 613–37; and my "Going Gently into That Good Night: A Review Essay on Callahan's *Setting Limits*," *Bioethics Books* 1, no. 1 (1989): 1–4. My "Measured Fairness, Situated Justice: Feminist Reflections on Health Care Rationing," *Kennedy Institute of Ethics Journal* 6, no. 1 (March 1996): 53–68, examines Kamm's and Daniels' work. Nancy S. Jecker's "Toward a Theory of Age-Group Justice," *Journal of Medicine and Philosophy* 14, no. 6 (1989): 655–76, takes on Daniels. See also Jecker's "Age-Based Rationing and Women," *Journal of the American Medical Association* 266 (1991): 3012–15.

11. Michael Neill, *Issues of Death: Morality and Identity in English Renaissance Tragedy* (New York: Oxford University Press, 1997). See also Terence Hawkes's review in the *London Review of Books* 19 (1997): 10–11, "On the Way in Which Tragedy 'Openeth up the Greatest Wounds and Showeth Forth the Ulcers That Are Covered with Tissue.'"

12. John Donne, "Death's Duel," in *Devotions upon Emergent Occasions Together with Death's Duel* (Ann Arbor: University of Michigan Press, 1959), 176–77, as quoted in Neill, *Issues of Death*, 11–12.

13. The philosophers of classical antiquity, who gave this question about death a good going over, seem to have been very interested in whether different ways of thinking and living could reduce the harm of death; see the discussion in Martha C. Nussbaum, *The Therapy of Desire: Theory and Practice in Hellenistic Ethics* (Princeton, N.J.: Princeton University Press, 1994). This is certainly a less developed tendency in contemporary discussions. See, however, Derek Parfit's "Should We Welcome or Regret My Conclusions?" in his *Reasons and Persons* (London: Oxford University Press, 1984). Kamm, as will be noted, is also interested in the possibility that developing certain virtues could make one less vulnerable to death's harms.

14. "Death" is probably most readily available in Thomas Nagel's *Mortal Questions* (Cambridge: Cambridge University Press, 1979).

15. Kamm probes many other possible ways in which death is bad. One on which she particularly focuses is the idea that death involves nothingness, which we regard as an "unexperienced bad." (See her discussion of "The Limbo Man" in chapters 1 and 3 of *Morality, Mortality.*) That we do so is shown by certain thought experiments that converge on the distinctive negativity of things being all over for us. This "Extinction Factor" Kamm regards as the most distinctive feature of our concern with death. But, on her own showing, death involves things being all over for us only in some (albeit crucial) respects. What is clearly all over is our access to the goods of experience and action.

16. Kamm, *Morality, Mortality*, 17. She points out that one finds unexperienced harms in death as well—for instance, a person might find death harmful because it truncated her chances of living so as to attract the admiration of future generations.

17. Kamm, *Morality, Mortality*, 61.

18. Nagel, *Mortal Questions*, 10.

19. Harold Pinter, *Moonlight* (New York: Dramatists Play Services, 1995), 13. Another way of seeing the particular poignancy of Andy's position is to see him now trying to reorient his sense of the worth of what he has accomplished, identifying himself not with specific accomplishments but with a structure that resists mortality—the "temple of the just." I don't think that the rhetorical failures of Andy's declamation—its bombast, for instance—represent flaws in Pinter. Rather, they suggest the failure of Andy's life, and the futility of his retrospective attempt to infuse it with lasting value.

20. Margaret Walker, *Moral Understandings: A Feminist Study in Ethics* (New York: Routledge, 1998), chapter 6.

21. Cheshire Calhoun, "Justice, Care, Gender Bias," *Journal of Philosophy* 85, no. 9 (September 1998): 451–63.

22. See Marilyn Frye's discussion of the "arrogant eye of masculine perception," in her "In and Out of Harm's Way," from *The Politics of Reality* (Trumansburg, N.Y.: Crossings Press, 1983), 66–72.

23. I don't mean to suggest that these notions are only interpretable in ways that stress the significance of experience and action. It is not only in the East that there are eschatological traditions that are contemplative or mystical, and not much interested in the survival of one's personality. However, here again is a point where Calhoun's insight is helpful—what is logically entailed by a theory can be overshadowed in philosophical importance by what is ideologically enacted.

24. About the therapeutic task of philosophy, I again cite Nussbaum's *Therapy of Desire*. Callahan powerfully inveighs against the notion that medicine will someday cure us of all our ills, including mortality, in book after book; *False Hopes* (New York: Simon & Schuster, 1998) continues the jeremiad.

5

"Everything Includes Itself in Power"
Power, Theory, and the Foundations of Bioethics

Then everything includes itself in power
Power into will, will into appetite;
And appetite, an universal wolf,
So doubly seconded with will and power,
Must make perforce an universal prey,
And last eat up himself.

William Shakespeare, *Troilus and Cressida*, Act One, Scene Three

A way of understanding an important theme in the history of ethics, at least since the Enlightenment, is to see it as an attempt to chain Shakespeare's universal wolf. Somehow, power must be kept from dissolving without residue into will and appetite. Otherwise, we run the risk of various kinds of war, which few regard as an efficient way of achieving their ends, and fewer still desire for its own sake. Further, we lose what strikes me as a deep human hope: that there are ways of living that are *legitimate*. By "legitimate" I mean that the circumstances and projects that form our lives are not merely expressions of a purely contingent play of historical forces with which we will have to either put up if we must or pull down if we can. Rather, we hope that our lives can be made to reflect, even if darkly, something that is true about the way things ought to be, in a way that, finally and fundamentally, is more than a matter of whatever you or I or anyone else might think or wish. The way things ought to be, according to this hope, will at least constrain and perhaps even guide our power, turning it to ends other than whatever we or others just might happen to desire, steering it toward what in fact we should yearn for. Should this hope fail, we face not only Hobbes' prospect of the war of each against all, but an even more profound threat: the loss of a deeply important fea-

89

ture of our notion of ourselves as agents. For if there is only power, and only will and appetite to guide it, if there is nothing to be said for any goal or guide or form of life that would distinguish it as more worth attending to than any other, then what is to prevent us from slipping into a kind of inertness, in which all pursuits are comparatively indifferent, and any pursuit seems ultimately vain? The will, as David Wiggins has noted, craves objective reasons in determining what is worth striving for: "often it could not go forward unless it thought it had them."[1]

Bioethics centrally concerns power—the power of technology and the power of healers. But what has bioethics to do with such issues as whether the will has objective moral reasons? Isn't it focused resolutely on a specific form of human practice, on the concerns of people other than professional philosophers, people who have to make real-time decisions in a real-time world? What has bioethics to do with metaethics, or metaethics with bioethics, for that matter?

It's in the impact that our power can have on our reasons that an answer to this natural question emerges. If the thought that our norms are based solely on the thin air of desires—whether solely our own, or more-or-less commonly shared—isn't widely disturbing, that is because it is not deeply believed. People typically have confidence that their fundamental moral commitments track something beyond will and appetite. It's true that there are important streams of contemporary thought (and classical thought, too) that deny any such status to moral claims, but for all their academic force, they have not penetrated very far into most people's common practices of deliberations and assessment, at least most of the time. That's all to the good: moral commitments are supposed to do some fairly heavy lifting in social life, including at times providing us with reasons to sacrifice even what we most desire, or to resist even highly popular beliefs; Wiggins is on to something when he suggests that we need to have confidence that our convictions are up to the job. Academic skepticism about the objective force of moral reasons, based, say, on excessive fondness for the notion of "social construction" (quite indispensable in its own way), or on concerns that it's "queer" that a reason could be both objective and action guiding, are unlikely to unseat that confidence.[2]

What does have the potential to be more corrosive that any academic skepticism is contemporary medicine. Medicine's new powers put on the table questions that are in important ways unprecedented, that are plainly crucial for the way in which our shared and our individual lives will go on, and which in some measure we cannot avoid, either as individuals or as members of a society. Just because those questions are so insistent, significant, distinctive, deep, and difficult, they threaten to expose the pervasive character of our moral pluralism, driving home the idea that our moral differences are rationally unbridgeable, and nurturing the thought that our failure here exposes our ethical commitments as either merely preferences that emerge from some combination of socialization and biology, or as deliverances that God has seen fit to give to us, but not to the heathen. As the seemingly intractable debates over abortion and other reproductive issues indicate, bioethical disputes can not only expose the moral fissures latent in our societies—they can excavate them more deeply.

Bioethics has to deal with some pretty conspicuous and controversial forms of power—power to predict who will sicken and die, and when and how they will do so; power to snatch from death's cusp. Power as well to avoid conception and birth, and to give children to the barren. One of its jobs is to craft reasonable regulations for the use of all this power. What is less clearly appreciated, though, is that these powers not only change our bodies, what they will suffer, and what they can do—they change our societies, our relationships, even our aspirations and values. They call into question what we owe one another, and why, and challenge us to forge new understandings of how we can go on together—or, at least, tolerably together—in the face of these new abilities, and the new disagreements they foster. They push us not only to deploy our moral resources in new ways, but to reexamine and renew those resources—to think metaethically, as well as ethically. And that, too, is a job for bioethics.

For the past three decades, scholars have been trying to figure out how to think carefully about what to do with all this power, about how to justify various ways of creating it, directing it, withholding it, paying for it. The options that have seemed most available to bioethics theorists fall into two broad camps. One approach is to try to find morally useful notions—rules, principles, stories, analogies, virtues—which will resonate with the many kinds of moral understandings that make up the "common morality." Thus, the popularity of beneficence and respect for autonomy as moral principles: they appeal to (virtually) all of us, although for very different reasons. What remains painfully unclear is how moral understandings that the going moral traditions share at this level of abstraction can be articulated to provide equally widely attractive resolutions to what are quite literally life and death problems.

The other approach is to try to find some moral ideals which can be vindicated by what might be called "pure" reason—not, that is, by clarifying the evaluative traditions prevalent in this or that form of life, but by demonstrating the inescapability of certain norms to all who count as rational agents.

The chief aim of this chapter is to try to support the first approach indirectly, by way of an extended critical analysis of an important instance of the second. I will be looking at one of the most theoretically sophisticated efforts to provide bioethics with a rationally inevitable starting point—the work of H. Tristram Engelhardt, as expressed in the second edition of *The Foundations of Bioethics*. The point of this exercise may seem a bit obscure—surely, Engelhardt's work, for all its formidable scholarship and intellectual power, stands out like a sore thumb: most bioethical theorists locate themselves in some corner of the first camp. Yet, while I certainly agree that Engelhardt's work fails, it is, I think, an instructive failure. For one reason, its aspirations to vindicate indisputably at least some constraints on power chime with what I have tried to portray here as an important feature of being a morally serious, reflective agent—the quest for legitimacy—in a way that takes very seriously indeed pluralism, the power of traditions, and the limits of reason. For another reason, Engelhardt is aware of how issues in bioethics show how the moral gaps that divide us pose such a serious problem for social life. Seeing how he goes wrong will be useful for, among other things, raising the question of whether the quest for legitimacy, in the face of the hard moral questions poised by technological advance in medicine, can be achieved using the resources of a less theoretically ambitious form of bioethical thinking.

I have a second rationale. Engelhardt's approach entails answers to our bioethical (and more broadly ethical) problems that strike me as frankly shocking. They constitute, as I see it, conclusions that morally serious people are not likely to be able to endorse unless they are enchanted by a theory. Hence, I aim also at disenchantment.

*   *   *

We think hard about how to live our lives, and we try to get it right. What keeps this enormously difficult job from being a vain passion? For Engelhardt, the world and our strivings in it are redeemed from ultimate vanity by God, who speaks with relative clarity to Orthodox Catholics, more obscurely to other Christians, more obscurely still to non-Christian believers, and altogether unintelligibly to many of us. Because, as Engelhardt acknowledges, God has not chosen to make the truth plain to all, many of the goals sought and constraints observed by Orthodox Catholics will seem, to one extent or another, undermotivated, confused, misunderstood, regrettable, perverse, or even evil, and any exercise of power in these directions will seem, insofar as it affects a nonbeliever such as me, more or less alien and arbitrary. Orthodox Catholics will, of course, have similar views about how I live my life, and the same problem will, mutatis mutandis, confront all of us.

So, at least as regards our social lives in a pluralist state, we all hear the howl of Shakespeare's wolf. Engelhardt's work stands in a long tradition of efforts to forge out of reason a chain for power. "A goal of ethics," he tells us, "is to determine when force can be justified."[3] But it is a tradition that, at least as he and many others see it, is just about out of gas. The idea that we could somehow find out how to domesticate the wolf, direct our power, appetite, and will toward ends that were (demonstrably) really good in ways that were (evidently) really right, relying for those demonstrations and that evidence on the exercise of faculties common to all persons, is not only unlikely in fact, but, according to Engelhardt, impossible in principle. Human reason has no canonical vision of how we all should live tucked away in its hat. Reason might help us better understand the implications of some constellation of normative commitments we accept on other grounds, set them in better, more perspicuous, more coherent order. But it cannot provide us with a guaranteed-to-be-correct transcendental blueprint of the good life. Nor, apparently, can it even justify the selection of plausible contenders for that role.

Any such blueprints as we have are the result of our participation in traditions much more specific than the point of view of reason as such, traditions that come with more-or-less rich conceptions of what is worth living for already installed. Within such traditions—with our "moral friends"—reason may be useful in the role of underlaborer, helping resolve unclarity or disagreement about what a tradition's vision of the good requires. Between one tradition and the next, however, there is grave disagreement concerning the good, and reason cannot resolve them.

What reason can do on its own, however, is justify rigorously a few minimal, but at the same time quite far-reaching, constraints on both our actions and our motivations. Roughly, Engelhardt takes reason as competent to demonstrate the following: we must not act in ways that involve other people without their permission (the permission principle), and we must be motivated to act in ways that seek the good of others, although what such motivation will concretely involve—what really constitutes the good of others—is impossible to specify outside the context of certain conceptions of the good that are not themselves determinable by reason (the principle of beneficence).[4]

A world in which the interactions among moral traditions were constrained only by these principles would not be so much a society as a nightmare. It would, for example, be a world in which a Canadian-style system of guaranteed access to health care would be seen as so coercive as to be immoral.[5] That, however, is a comparatively trivial consequence. In Engelhardt's world, toddlers as well as veal calves could be fattened for the table in factory farms. Our desire to witness violence would not have to be sublimated via football, but could be more robustly gratified by the spectacle of gladiators hacking each other to death. All that would be needed to put such modest proposals into practice, apart from a good deal of money, is the permission of the morally considerable parties to these practices, bolstered by assurances that the motivations involved were not flat-out malevolent.[6] In the world ordered by Engelhardt's permission principle, toddlers are not morally considerable; they can neither extend permission to others to do anything, nor regulate their own behavior according to permissions granted. Even in our own world, all kinds of nonmalevolent motivations for blood sports can be offered: they sharpen the eye, make a nice day out with friends, enact and deepen old traditions. The upshot is that if parents wanted to sell their infants, and promoters could attract contestants, a market in baby meat and gladiatorial games would have to be tolerated.

Nor is this all. The same kind of horrors stem from the stringency of the permission principle, as from its laxity, coupled with the emptiness of the beneficence principle. It would always be blameworthy, Engelhardt says, to kill one innocent, unconsenting person, even if failure to do so caused the deaths of billions. What he doesn't say, but which seems just as strictly implied by his position, is that it would never be permissible merely to nudge an unconsenting, innocent person slightly to the left, if that were somehow the necessary condition required to avert mass destruction. The assessment that the supposed catastrophe were worse than inconveniencing an unconsenting, innocent person would necessarily draw upon certain rationally undemonstrable and, in the present case, unshared ideas of how certain outcomes should be valued, and hence, could not confer secular moral authority.[7]

While sincerely lamenting the poverty of its implications, Engelhardt is still a true fan of the methodology of modern philosophy. Not for him are the tempered ambitions of many contemporary mainstream moral theorists—including most of his bioethical colleagues—who incline to the view that achieving coherence among our principles, our best conceptions of the world overall, and our considered moral judgments lends reasonableness, and perhaps even warrant, to those judgments.[8] His ethics will have a rationally unassailable foundation; it doesn't matter that no one can live in the structure it supports.

Engelhardt's basic motivation is that there is simply no ranking of goods for which reasons can be given of a kind that would show anyone who rejected them to be irrational. If we attempted to shut down the baby slaughterhouses, or even shove a recalcitrant gentleman to his left to spare the rest of creation, without such reasons at our disposal, we would be guilty of what is virtually the only thing we can know (in a publicly defensible way) to be a moral enormity: treating persons—or, more precisely, innocent persons—in ways in which they have not in some significant way consented.

As a good foundationalist, Engelhardt spends much of his book displaying the implications of his view for particular problems in bioethics; for the most part, his resolutions cohere closely with his fundamental philosophical commitments. But, learned, thoughtful, and imaginative though it be, this is not the feature of his work that will engage my interest here. The core of my critique concerns Engelhardt's attempt to demonstrate that the permission principle is binding on all rational agents insofar as they would be moral.

ENGELHARDT'S TRANSCENDENTAL DEDUCTION

In the crucial second chapter of the *Foundations*, Engelhardt categorizes the possible ways in which one might provide general secular reasons for moral conclusions, and finds them all wanting. No such reasons will ever be able to show how we ought to live our lives in any detail; we cannot know on such grounds what we ought to strive for, what we should attempt to avoid, what is noble, what base, or what we are to make of our dependence on others, and theirs on us. The answers to such questions reside in specific moral traditions, whose adherents may well share the kind of commitments to a notion of the good that can both guide a life and make thinking about morality profitable. As Engelhardt thinks, some of the answers to be found in such communities are true (Orthodox Catholicism), some false (those of every other community insofar as they disagree with Orthodox

Catholicism), and some simply incoherent (cosmopolitan yuppies, who survive off an ill-fitting, badly understood, and unsupported mélange of Judeo-Christian moral precepts which cannot be justified outside the metaphysical commitments of those religious views). But all are rationally indemonstrable.

It might seem bold to claim that it can be known that no effort to rationally assess, refute, reform, or justify the moral understandings of the traditions or quasi-traditions in which we find ourselves could ever be successful. But Engelhardt's argument is forceful. In essence, he claims that whatever system of normative justification you favor—intuitionistic, casuistical, consequentialist, rational choice, game theoretic, natural law, or what have you—will always presuppose the very thing it is trying to justify: a particular moral understanding, in terms of which intuitions, cases, consequences, and so forth assume their moral salience. Consider, for instance, Engelhardt's critique of intuitionism. He generates examples that bring home both the conflict in intuitions among moral agents, and the fact that the intuitions of a given agent may underdetermine the choices she faces. How can we resolve these conflicts without relying on some notion of the good for which intuitionism cannot itself account? In considering consequentialist approaches, Engelhardt points out that theoretical options within that family of views will also always involve some commitment to values for which the theories cannot account. Should we be hedonic or agathistic utilitarians? Average or total consequentialists? What discount rate should we use in considering the impact of actions on the future? Appealing to "the consequences" obviously can't sort out these questions, since what they all come down to is just what "appealing to the consequences" is going to mean. The theory seems incapable of resolving these issues without drawing on the resources of some sense of value it presupposes, rather than vindicates.

Engelhardt presses the same kind of point against other standard approaches relentlessly. This is not to say that he leaves not a stone upon a stone: intuitionists, for instance, might reply that the existence of disagreement and underdetermination among agents does not by itself show that there are no intuitions generally recognized as having moral authority; implications for unclear cases might be teased out analogically, not in a way that guarantees apodictic certainty, but which yields strong presumptions for or against other courses of action and understanding. Utilitarians, for example, might choose to maximize preferences rather than pleasure, happiness, or interests, precisely in order to sidestep making general normative commitments, locating these outside the theory, in individuals. But it surely isn't clear that any of these moves would be successful against Engelhardt's critique. Preferences as such may simply leave me cold; I may have epistemological views that make the prospect of relying on an intuition ridiculous. Yet however it stands with general proofs of the categorical impossibility of ever demonstrating the correctness of a particular system of moral justification, it surely must be granted that disagreement about these matters in the present state of knowledge need not escape the bounds of what is rational.

However, despite the fact that no "content-full" moral notion is generally available, we are not, as Engelhardt sees it, reduced altogether to moral nihilism in our dealings with those who do not share our particular view. There remains the permission principle (his principle of beneficence is too vacuous to do much work between moral strangers). Even in the face of reason's failure to defend any content-full notion of morality, we can still morally guide interchanges among strangers in terms of what they have agreed to, and hence, at least thus far, chain the wolf.

Engelhardt takes on a pretty stiff epistemic burden in defending this view; his own positions have to be insulated against the skeptical strategy he advances against the standard accounts—a strategy which largely amounts to pointing out that there are serious arguments against accepting any of those views. One might say, for example, that he has an analogous problem with "future discount rates" to that with which he has taxed consequentialists; do my agreements (i.e., mutual conferrals of permissions upon others and theirs upon me) bind me as stringently twenty years after they are made as they do now? He seems to incline to the view that they do, but there are contrary positions. Derek Parfit, for example, thinks that promises made in the distant past are less binding than those recently made, alerting us to how the whole matter may rest on very complex and contestable issues in the theory of identity over time.[9]

Other questions suggest themselves. Am I to regard all agreements, no matter what turns out to be the consequences of keeping them, as equally sacrosanct? Or do agreements come in different flavors, from the profound to the trivial? (For obvious reasons, the answer to these questions cannot itself be simply a matter of what some people happen to agree to.) Certainly, some of my authoritative agreements are tacit—Engelhardt says as much in his analysis of the justification of adolescent children remaining under the authority of their parents.[10] Mightn't it be said that my agreement not to engage in buying or sell-ing luxury health care in Ontario, or to put up an English sign over my business in Quebec, is tacitly given by my continued residence in such places? The police of neither government will hinder me from leaving, after all. What, then, are the limits to implicit agreements? Why, for example, should I pay any attention to the distribution of property I encounter as I emerge into awareness of the social conventions of my society? That distribution affects my life in major ways, I did not explicitly agree to it, and even if current distributions could be understood in terms of free agreements (an enormously dubious idea) there seems little reason to regard the Lockean view of property Engelhardt apparently accepts as itself true beyond the possibility of a reasonable doubt.[11]

General answers to many of these questions emerge out of Engelhardt's text, but it is surely inviting to imagine that many of them involve a certain understanding of the value of keeping commitments that is presupposed in his version of the view, not justified by it. Or, as in the case of his views of personal identity and the analysis of property, they rest on other, eminently contestable philosophical views.

I propose, however, to refrain from examining metaphysical issues concerning how best to understand just what these persons are who make long-term agreements, or what is the limit of their decision-making authority, and try to take seriously Engelhardt's claim that the permission view does not stem from any notion that "permission"—or "persons," for that matter—has any particular moral value (as any such assignment to these notions of moral value would be contestable and indemonstrable).

Engelhardt claims that, in the free agreements of "moral strangers"—those who do not share a given moral tradition—we see disclosed "a transcendental condition of the possibility of a general domain of human life and of the life of persons generally . . . [namely, the domain composed of] speaking of blame and praise with moral strangers, and . . . establishing a particular set of moral commitments with an authority other than through force."[12] Although Engelhardt refers to this domain as "unavoidable,"[13] the nature of the imperative involved in taking a moral point of view seems distinctly hypothetical. He allows that the moral authority of free agreements requires a decision to collaborate. So the position actually seems to be the following: if we wish to interact with others on terms other than those of force, then we need to see our agreements with them as possessing moral authority.

I take the invocation of "moral authority" to mean something of this sort: even if it turned out subsequent to my making such an agreement that it did not serve my interests, and even if it were the case that I could fail to adhere to the agreement in a way that would make me better off (for example, circumstances in which I could depart from the agreement undetectably), I should still adhere to the agreement.

Now, why ever should I do that?

My question is not a version of the "Why should I be moral?" chestnut. What I am asking is this: what in the desiccated world with which Engelhardt leaves us, makes according with agreements moral, and reneging on them, immoral? What is there in what Engelhardt has said which would provide me with anything that I could rationally count as a moral reason—a secular, public kind of moral reason—for sticking to an agreement? One answer that springs quickly to mind is that doing so will be more likely to preserve a peaceable community than not doing so. Engelhardt, however, is very explicit that this is not *his* reason—"This view of ethics and bioethics is not grounded in a concern for peaceableness," he writes.[14] While it may be true that accordance with commitments will tend to preserve peaceable communities, one could only see that as a reason for action against a backdrop that put a positive value on such communities, and, as Engelhardt sees it, there's no secular ground for thinking that any such view is more reasonable than views that despise peaceable communities, that see divergence in moral understandings as the perfect pretext for the exercise of the heroic virtues that only conflict can nurture. Some may well prefer to kill the infidel, even if that means pulling the temple down on top of their own heads, too.[15]

Another possible candidate for a reason here is that securing a reliable way of arranging terms of cooperation with others apart from force should be very attractive to any agent. I have excellent reason to believe that, whatever it is that I value, in the long run I will be more likely to obtain it if peaceable, reliable, coordinated action with others is a standard feature of life. Accordingly, I act irrationally if I do that which undermines peaceable coordination. But this reason still leaves me thinking strategically rather than morally: if I am very powerful, or extremely subtle, or know I will die soon anyway, then it may well be very much an open question whether it is in my long-term best interests to, say, keep my word, or to avoid violence. The key here is my prudential judgment about the impact of my departure from the standing terms, and, as I am confident Engelhardt would say, what constitutes prudence here is unintelligible apart from my adherence to a rationally underdetermined sense of what is good.

The straw still floating at this point seems to be the idea that it is necessary that I regard my agreements as authoritative and keep to them (or, at least, see myself as bound by them, and recognize that I am a worthy target of censure and other blame if I renege) if I am appropriately to describe my relationships to others as moral. In other words, standing by my agreements simply is what it is to act morally (as this notion is understandable in secular contexts). This seems to me closest to what Engelhardt means in this chapter. But it also is unlikely to keep the wolf from the door, for it seems a purely stipulative use of "moral." Apart from strategic considerations, it is curious indeed why anyone advantageously positioned would see herself as having any reason to care about whether her conduct is so describable. If there's nothing more behind it than Engelhardt has yet shown us, then "morality" is just a word.

In sum, then, my criticism of Engelhardt is this: in relegating morality (in the secular realm) to a matter of coordinating various kinds of permission-giving and agreement-keeping among those able to give permission and make agreements, devoid of any resources for explaining what it is about the ability of persons to permit and agree that ought to command our respect (since any such account would draw on some content-full, and therefore unjustifiable, conception of the value of persons and their deeds), it seems impossible to understand how permissions and agreements, as such, count as moral reasons for action.

As this point is so central to understanding and assessing what Engelhardt is up to in *Foundations*, and as the critical reply I here make to his position seems so natural, I want to spend some further time trying to understand how the viewpoint expressed in the permission principle could reasonably have moral authority. I'll consider two possibilities. One concerns Engelhardt's attempt to analogize his notion of the conditions for the possibility of moral discourse with conditions for the possibility of empirical enquiry. The other has to do with the possibility that those moral strangers who meet together to resolve what Engelhardt does, after all, call moral problems, all bring just the kind of understanding of what morality is at base so as to fit with unique snugness into his framework.

THE ANALOGY WITH SCIENCE

In his third chapter, Engelhardt writes:

> The concrete fabric of morality must then be based on a will to a moral viewpoint. . . . The secular moral point of view . . . will be that intellectual standpoint from which one understands that conflicts regarding the propriety or impropriety of a particular action can be resolved intersubjectively by mutual agreement, and which viewpoint one then embraces in order to enable an intersubjectively grounded practice of blaming and praising, of mutual respect, and of moral authority. The moral fabric sustaining the various forms of the moral life is then a general practice that is as unavoidable as is the interest in resolving moral disputes. In terms of that morality, mutual respect becomes understood as using others only with their permission.[16]

One way of understanding this passage is to see it as signaling Engelhardt's resignation of yet another of the traditional hopes of moral philosophy: providing good reasons why we should take up a moral point of view at all. The suggestion seems to be that morality depends on the will, not the intellect—on a "will to a moral viewpoint" that is motivated, so I suppose, by nothing other than the attractiveness of morality itself. But invoking the autonomy of morality is not the problem. The problem is that what the will is supposed to light upon in seeking a moral point of view—the binding force of agreement—is not even an intelligible candidate for that role without some further reason for thinking that agreements with persons ought to be kept for reasons that go beyond mere prudence.

Engelhardt's talk of "enabling blaming or praising," of "mutual respect" and "moral authority" is unhelpful. He may indeed be describing a language game in which such phrases as "you are to blame" can be appropriately used only in relation to a person's behavior with respect to another person's agreements, and in which notions of authority and respect are also defined in these terms. But there is no reason given for thinking that we should invest these phrases with anything like the importance that we do in our ordinary contexts of moral discourse. When I blame someone for breaking a promise, this makes sense because promise breaking, in the absence of very serious reasons of certain restricted kinds, expresses contempt, or at least insufficient respect, toward beings I regard as worthy of respect in virtue of their value and vulnerabilities. For Engelhardt, blaming someone for breaking an agreement seems to involve marking their failure to respect another being who is worthy of respect solely in virtue of their being able to make agreements. While my account surely needs to be filled in, Engelhardt's seems to have nowhere to go.

Engelhardt claims that his principle of respect for permission is somehow analogous to accepting the principle of induction to ground empirical knowledge claims. I understand this claim along the following lines. Suppose someone were to say, "The sun will rise in the east tomorrow," and cite for evidence the fact that it always has done before. Imagine a skeptic replying, "Look, that it has done so before is absolutely no evidence that it will in the future. What you really need here is some metaphysical claim to the regularity of nature. But apart from special revelation from God, we know that there is no reason to believe that any such argument will ever succeed; Hume showed that. So this claim about the sun is completely unsupported." From what I can make out, Engelhardt thinks the appropriate response to the skeptic's reply should run this way: assuming the regularity of nature is simply part of what it is to make an empirical generalization, a condition of the possibility of this region of discourse, or something of that sort.

So the analogy here is supposed to be, just as making an empirical generalization presupposes induction, making a secular moral assessment presupposes the permission principle. But the analogy limps. Whatever might be said about the ultimate bona fides of induction, clearly a minimally coherent life presupposes some degree of regularity; we simply are not at liberty, in any practical sense, to act as though we did not believe that the past was at all relevant as a guide to the present. And, as a matter of fact, we do believe it: I see no reason to think that acceptance of the idea that the future will resemble the past in ways we can identify and project is not an essential part of commonsense metaphysics. But with moderate effort, a person can imagine, and (with rather more effort) even live, a life in which her relationships with moral strangers were not moral in any ordinary sense, nor even in the Engelhardtian sense of granting nonstrategic authority to agreements. One might be perfectly strategic about the whole matter, acting in accord with one's agreements insofar as one had self-interested reasons for doing so, and not otherwise; international relations gives us a good view of this way of conducting a life writ large.

We could, then, make agreements with moral strangers, and respect each others' extendings and withholdings of permissions in the manner of an enlightened egoist. We might even agree to arrange things in the world to make respecting permissions and agreements more likely to be in one's own interest. I'd be very happy not to call the resulting system a moral one, but it is far from being impossible. If one gives up the necessary conditions for the very coherence of the physical world, one has given up on sanity. If one has given up on Engelhardt's candidate for a necessary condition for the very coherence of the moral world (insofar as it involves strangers)—the principle of permission—you've got plenty left. In addition, of course, there seems no reason to accept that such a "moral world," erected on such a slender and unlovely basis, has anything attractive enough about it that we should worry about its coherence, unless it is its promise of avoiding conflict. But that, of course, may not always matter to us. And it may not always be at issue.

THE RELATIONSHIP BETWEEN SECULAR AND CONTENT-FULL MORALITIES

Perhaps what I have regarded as unjustifiable stealing from the forbidden territory of content-full moral views is not at all illicit on Engelhardt's view. Perhaps what he really thinks is that our motivation to be moral stems from our diverse repositories of moral content, and that, in coming to disagreements with strangers with a community-based motivation to avoid conflict and do what there are good reasons to do, or something of that sort, we come to realize on reflection that the only features of our moral commitments that survive the acid skepticism of postmodernity are those which can be expressed in the principle of permission. On this reading, I will keep my agreements with Engelhardt for roughly Kantian reasons, and he will keep his with me because God so commands, but when we meet as strangers, we leave behind both Kant and God and merely keep a sense of the moral seriousness of agreements with others.

But little seems to be gained by this move. Recall that we want secular morality to be able to lend some principled, defensible coordination to human life. For example, the state is empowered to enforce contracts, and its coercions here are supposed to be justified by reason. But on the interpretation we are now considering, the moral warrant for the coercive enforcement of agreements is not simply the permission principle as it may be understood in a secular light; it is a permission principle which is motivated by what might be called an overlapping consensus among the partisans of many content-full moralities. But ultimately, no secular reason can be given for accepting any of the content-full moralities that motivate secular allegiance to the permission principle; hence, there ultimately is no secular reason that permits coercion of those who dissent. It is, after all, false to think that everyone is going to regard all agreements and permissions as equally morally authoritative, albeit on distinct and incommensurate grounds; some may not regard them as morally significant at all. Many others will regard them as having some kind of moral authority, but not in ways that cohere with Engelhardt's understanding of their form and force. On its own terms, then, the secular moral world as envisaged by Engelhardt acts wrongly if it acts coercively toward those who do not accept the permission principle, and it cannot be assumed that all will, or even—in their own terms—that they should.

Try as I may, then, I cannot see how to invest the permission principle with the magic Engelhardt sees for it. Apart from some no doubt contestable belief that people matter morally, it is hard to grasp why their agreements should.

APRÈS MOI, LE DELUGE?

If the permission principle, understood as a delivery of transcendental reason, lacks any kind of moral authority worth caring about, then it is vain to attempt to understand it in that fashion anymore. All it reflects, then, is a specific understanding of what is of value in human lives; hence, the permission principle slips back into the pack with all the other attempts to make sense of ourselves as moral agents. It seems to me important to acknowledge that it does so; apart from the philosophical imperative of trying to get straight about such things for their own sakes, the permission principle—at least hooked up with certain views of property acquisition with which it is often associated and which Engelhardt seems quite willing to espouse—will generally tend to justify distributions of power in private hands in their present, highly inegalitarian fashion. If this is morally justifiable, then it will have to be shown to be so in contrast with other competing, content-full notions of justice, and not handed the palm because of some claim to a unique form of rational grounding. Reason is not guiding power here; indeed, it looks much more as though we have yet another instance of power gobbling reason up.

But this returns us to Engelhardt's skepticism. Without his transcendental Archimedean point, have we any way of engaging in moral discourse with those who do not share our traditions? And, to my mind, an even more disturbing question follows hard on: absent good reasons, have we any way of understanding why we ourselves should espouse our own traditions, particularly if we lack faith that their truth is guaranteed by God?

Engelhardt's concern is that all the ways that people make sense of and direct their lives involve commitment to values and to rankings of values that are widely various among individuals, communities, cultures, traditions, and so forth. All attempts to rationally justify any of these systems simply assume what is to be proved, and hence are useless, except perhaps as devices to explicate a given vision. As universal conversion to any specific tradition is not a realistic hope, and as there can be no argument proving that people should accept the aspirations and constraints of any tradition, there can be no moral authority outside the communities informed by given traditions, either. The play of power is all that we can rely upon in public space.

This strikes me as a fear that is motivated by the same hope that the Enlightenment bred: in the absence of transcendental grounds of some sort for constraints on our behavior, anything goes. A view from nowhere, or blindness. If God is dead, all is permitted. It seems to me that we needn't live on such dramatic heights. Rather, we can approach the task of making sense of, refining, and even justifying the moral understandings by which we live immanently, rather than transcendentally. We must start from where we are, elucidating what we value, relating our various commitments, striving for greater coherence among our moral, philosophical, and empirical beliefs, regarding disagreements with others, insofar as we can, as chances to increase the power and scope of our own understandings. We need to balance allegiance to our moral commitments with an awareness of our fallability, and hence of their revisability. We need to attend to our best ideas about what makes a person a good and discerning moral judge, sensitive to the highly nuanced forms in which our values combine to provide reasons for certain responses, and to the extreme sensitivity of moral reasons to context. This is, of course, is an impressionistic sketch of a wide reflective equilibrium approach to moral justification, amplified by concerns about what is sometimes called "ethical formation."[17]

Would this sort of a practice, even in ideal terms, ever leave us any better off in terms of the rationality of our moral beliefs? Would it ever put us in a position where we could close the baby-abattoirs, call a halt to the gladiatorial games, or even tax citizens in service of a schedule of goods with which they may not fully agree—universal health care, for example, or federal funding for human embryonic stem cell research—and not simply be ravening the slaughterhouse owners, the eager gladiators, or the dissenting citizens, Shakespeare's universal wolf striking yet again?

The project of postmodernity is to make sense of reason in the face of our confinement to the circle of this world; this is a project that faces us in science, as much as it does in ethics. If we are to understand our judgments, be they moral, empirical, or conceptual, as nonarbitrary—and it is essential to our continuing to make sense of ourselves as rational agents that we do so—we will have to understand "nonarbitrariness" immanently. This, I think, may be most difficult for thinkers such as Engelhardt, who have allegiance to a very robust notion of the transcendental, and who see the postmodern condition, I suspect, as a function of the Fall. But it isn't easy for any of us, particularly as new powers, drawn primarily from the life sciences, push hard against some of our most settled notions of how to live well, and leave many of us on different sides of deep divides. If there's a text from which we may take some heart, it may be the trenchant observation with which Derek Parfit concludes his *Reasons and Persons*: nonreligious moral philosophy is a very young study. The complaint that it has failed to provide us with decisive and evidently warranted ways of living and understanding, with an unbreakable chain for the wolf, may be as premature as an analogous complaint would have been had it been lodged against the science of the eighteenth century.

If, however, disciplined reflection about morality is to provide us with such a chain, we shouldn't expect it to do so in a way that is more intellectually persuasive than has been achieved by the most advanced science of the twenty-first century. We don't get, and don't need, unassailable foundations or apodictic certainty there. Rather, we find within progressive, fallibilist, open traditions of inquiry, good reasons on which to rest our beliefs. To the extent we can achieve in bioethics what we've achieved in biology, we'll have achieved quite enough to be getting on with.

ACKNOWLEDGMENTS

I'm grateful for Brendan Minogue's invitation to lecture to the conference, "Ethics, Medicine and Health Care: An Appraisal of the Thought of H. Tristram Engelhardt," and, of course, to Professor

Engelhardt himself for his inspiring commitment to scholarship, and still more for his penchant for playing the foil to perfection. Philip Boyle graciously loaned me his home on the Hudson when I was between houses; on his sunny deck, poised between the river and Sing-Sing, the thoughts here started to take shape. Hilde Lindemann Nelson patiently read several versions, each time to my advantage.

NOTES

1. David Wiggins, "Truth, Invention, and the Meaning of Life," *Proceedings of the British Academy* (1976), reprinted in his *Needs, Values, Truth* (Oxford: Basil Blackwell and the Aristotelian Society, 1987), where the quote appears on p. 341. For discussion, see James Lindemann Nelson, "Desire's Desire for Moral Realism: A Phenomenological Objection to Noncognitivism," *Dialogue* 28 (1989): 449–60.

2. A classic source of the notion that "objective moral facts" would be ontologically "queer" entities, in that they would need to have properties necessary to exist independently of our wills, and also properties required to exert influence on our wills, is J. L. Mackie's *Ethics: Inventing Right and Wrong* (Hammondsworth: Penguin Books, 1977). A good critical discussion is contained in Sabina Lovibond, *Realism and Imagination in Ethics* (Minneapolis: University of Minnesota Press, 1983).

3. H. Tristram Engelhardt, Jr., *The Foundations of Bioethics*, 2nd ed. (Oxford and New York: Oxford University Press, 1996), 67.

4. See the discussion in *Foundations*, chapter 2, especially p. 67ff, and chapter 3. It may be worth noting that Engelhardt is committed to the view that acting does not include refraining. Otherwise, it would seem impossible not to act in ways that sometimes involve others without their permission.

5. As Engelhardt suggests on p. 385.

6. One could, for instance, justify consensual gladiatorial contests with reference to the "delectation" of the spectacle, and the "refined recall of the kill" with other fans of the game. See Engelhardt on hunting, *Foundations*, 141.

7. See p. 130 of *Foundations*. Engelhardt does say that it would be permissible to use deadly force against someone who was an innocent threat to my life. Is the key difference here that in the first case, I—the agent who alone could interfere with the threat—am not personally at risk of life and limb?

8. The image described is, of course, that of Rawls. For a manageable statement, see his "The Independence of Moral Theory," *Proceedings and Addresses of the American Philosophical Association* 48 (1974–1975). See also Norman Daniels, "Wide Reflective Equilibrium and Theory Acceptance in Ethics," *Journal of Philosophy* 76, no. 5 (1979), and Michael R. DePaul's *Balance and Refinement* (New York and London: Routledge, 1993). Tom

Beauchamp and James F. Childress endorse wide reflective equilibrium in chapter 9 of *The Principles of Biomedical Ethics* (New York: Oxford University Press, 2002, 5th edition). For the compatibility of a coherence methodology—of which reflective equilibrium may be seen as an instance—with a realist view about moral reasons, see David Brink, *Moral Realism and the Foundations of Ethics* (Cambridge: Cambridge University Press, 1983).

9. Derek Parfit, *Reasons and Persons* (Oxford: Oxford University Press, 1984).

10. Engelhardt, *Foundations*, 156.

11. See, for a relevant discussion, Clark Wolf, "Contemporary Property Rights, Lockean Provisos, and the Interests of Future Generations," *Ethics* 105, no. 4 (1995): 791–818.

12. Engelhardt, *Foundations*, 70.

13. Engelhardt, *Foundations*, 69.

14. Engelhardt, *Foundations*, 70.

15. Of course, such folks are choosing not to be moral in Engelhardt's terms (that is, in what he takes to be the only terms open to a secular morality), and thus opening themselves up for what he regards as the appropriate censure of rational beings from other parts of the universe, and the violent response of others. While one might well wish to avoid either response, that surely is different from seeing either as deserved. In other words, I might refrain from violating the permission principle if I feared the wrath of those I violated or the scorn of observing aliens. What seems unintelligible is refraining from living out my warrior ethic simply and solely because it violated the principle.

16. Engelhardt, *Foundations*, 104.

17. For some of the relevant amplification, see DePaul, cited in note 7; Jonathan Dancy, *Moral Reasons* (Oxford: Blackwells, 1993); and Sabina Lovibond, *Ethical Formation* (Cambridge, Mass.: Harvard University Press, 2002).

6

A Duty to Donate?
Selves, Societies, and Organ Procurement

In the latter part of the twentieth century, human bodies acquired what is widely seen as an unsettling new ability: their vital organs now have the power to sustain the lives of *other* human bodies. This new ability has extended the lives of tens of thousands of people around the world, providing the organs' recipients and those with whom they live with the potential for active, fulfilling years and continued rich relationships that otherwise would be denied them.

Alas, this new power has also spawned enormous difficulties. Some patients have found transplantation, or the associated burdens required to avoid rejecting their new organs, troublesome, unsatisfactory, or unsuccessful, so that little in the way of good quality extra time was provided at all, or was provided only at great cost. Social burdens have been considerable as well, although it is hard to calculate them accurately, since it is not clear what kind of opportunity costs transplantation medicine has extracted. Suppose we had devoted to primary care for inner city kids the resources earmarked for organ transplantation? More years of life saved, or fewer? Would medical, as opposed to surgical, responses to end-stage organ failure be further advanced had fewer of our resources and attention been directed to developing and improving transplantation? At the end of the day, might our enthusiasm for transplantation have actually resulted in a net loss of value?

These are tough questions. But there are aspects of organ transplantation just as disturbing as either its demonstrable or its speculative inefficiency as a means of extending human lives. The medical and social decision to invest so heavily in transplantation as a way of dealing with end-stage organ disease has forced us to make what Guido Calabresi and Philip Bobbit called in their celebrated book, *Tragic Choices,* "exposed choices against life."[1] It is notorious that the supply of transplantable organs persistently lags far behind the demand, with the result that society has had to cobble together a succession of elaborate rationing frameworks. These schemes are, of course, fair game for criticism by bioethicists, philosophers, and other scholars. More significantly perhaps, the fairness of prevailing allocation schemes has been challenged by public policy makers, by patients and families, and by citizens generally. This isn't surprising, as notions of what justice demands of us in distributing scarce, precious resources are complex, varied, and highly contested. But the disagreements are not solely matters for academic deliberation; insofar as potential donors, for example, find the allocation system unjust, they are the less likely to contribute to it, thus worsening the very problem the rationing system must try to solve.

To avoid, or at least relieve, the challenges of rationing, either demand must be reduced—scarcely likely in a time when transplant programs are increasingly willing and able to provide their services to people previously barred from consideration by reason of age or disease states—or supply increased. This chapter is about certain neglected moral issues involved in what might be called "supply-side" strategies.

The ground here is heavily trodden; the literature is full of discussions of the ethics of various plans aimed at increasing the availability of transplantable organs. However, I aim to travel this terrain in some different directions. I will ask whether the persistent difficulties in meeting the need for transplantable organs point to something more than glitches in how we advertise and promote donation, or natural and acceptable limits in the degree of altruism we can expect from people, particularly in the tragic circumstances in which organs are so often solicited. I also hope to guide attention away from the growing interest in turning human body parts into marketable commodities as a response to organ shortages. The fundamental question that will concern me here can be put this way: might this enduring pattern of allowing organs that could save human lives to molder uselessly away in dead bodies hint at deep moral flaws within our social arrangements?

I'll go at this question in a way that involves reimagining the new ability of parts of our bodies to sustain other people. I will propose that we see organ transplantation not merely as a technological tour de force, but as a pointed invitation to understand differently the character of our relationships to one another. Responses to the moral challenges posed by organ transplantation have taken entrenched moral and political understandings largely as given, and have attempted to fit various procurement and allocation schemes to prevailing normative notions. My aim here is to stand this approach on its head. Specifically, I will be arguing that our collective reluctance to provide more organs to those who need them reflects in some part those features of our culture that encourage us to think of ourselves, and of human goods, in too individualistic a fashion. Liberalism as a political philosophy, or, perhaps more accurately, as a political ideology, may bear some of the blame here, as may certain beliefs and anxieties bound up with certain normative understandings of gender roles. I will argue further that organ transplantation can reasonably be portrayed in ways that may help erode this kind of atomism; indeed, that it invites such portrayal. The image of organ transplantation I hope to make attractive can affiliate itself with less dominant, less aggressively individualistic moral understandings of social and political relationships in general, and in particular, lead to a better appreciation of what we owe each other as potential saviors of each others' lives.

ORGANS: METAPHORS AND MODELS

I've called the potential of sustaining other lives with the use of one's own organs a "new ability," but people for whom pregnancy has been an experience or is a prospect may not find it quite so novel—female bodies have, after all, always typically possessed a certain form of this ability. But the analogy with pregnancy—or, more accurately, "pregnability"—is not one that has been much invoked in discussions of human organ transplantation. We have not turned to characteristically female reproductive powers and the social meanings that accompany them, as a model for better understanding how we ought to live in the light of the new powers and relationships made possible by transplant technology. In fact, the chief acknowledgment of possible analogues between organ provision and pregnancy has moved in quite the opposite direction: it has been argued that since fathers, for instance, cannot be legally forced to provide organs, or even renewable tissues such as bone marrow, for their children, mothers should not be legally forced to provide their body to maintain the lives of fetuses that might become their children.

In the United States we have, rather, turned to metaphors of gift, construing the decision to make organs available or to withhold them as fundamentally a private matter, an expression of charity, rather than an expression of social solidarity; an outpouring of largesse, rather than a kind of care for the vulnerable that we have reasonable grounds to expect of each other. That "gift" rather than "gestation" has been the metaphor of choice may not, on reflection, seem odd: not only are there clearly disanologies between organ provision and pregnancy, but the meaning of pregnancy itself, and of the relationships between gravid women and the fetuses they harbor, is much contested. "Gift," in contrast, is a very commodious and not particularly contentious conceptual category. The psychic and social complexities of gifts are hidden by at least a surface agreement on what they are and what they mean. One might even say that it is not metaphoric at all to speak of organs made available for transplant as gifts; under the present dispensation, they are quite literally gifts, so concerns about disanologies are beside the point.

Yet, as I will try to show, thinking of organs as gifts occludes important moral considerations, despite the apparent transparency of the "gift" idea. In contrast, thinking of our ability to use our bodies to support the lives of others in ways influenced by ideas about pregnancy will bring these moral considerations to the fore, despite the limits of the pregnability metaphor. While the conceptual and moral issues involved with women's reproductive powers are complex, and women's right to control those abilities is of the first importance—indeed, this can scarcely be emphasized sufficiently—pregnancy and pregnability have discernable social and moral meanings that go beyond serving as a backdrop for disputes about whether and when women may choose to reject relationships.

At the level of a cultural theme—not to be confused with the level of individual psychology—the kind of intimate nurturing that pregnancy symbolizes is plausibly construed as one reason why femaleness has been associated with an image of rich and concrete human interconnectedness as the basic moral mise-en-scène, and with care and compassion as both natural tendencies and leading moral ideals. This contrasts with the more Hobbesian conceit associated with maleness: a sketch of a world within we must always keep our guard up and our self-interest centrally in view as we try to create somewhat precarious moral relationships with others. Individualism, self-reliance, and contractual relations are the guiding leitmotifs; care beyond contract is seen as wholly or largely discretionary, at least outside of the private sphere.

Some scholars—famously, Carol Gilligan—have argued that women and men do tend to employ different strategies of moral imagination and practical reasoning that reflect these patterns.[2] Yet it is important to stress that acknowledging the presence, power, and gendered associations of these themes is not necessarily to enter a claim about how real women and men always or even typically think about their lives and their relationships; there are surely plenty of women who rate independence from others very highly in their own conceptions of how best to live, plenty of men who cherish relationships intensely—and it's a good thing, too.

The notion, rather, is that such ideas as "connectedness," "relationship," and "caring" tend to cluster both together, and with the idea of femaleness, or perhaps with the feminine, much as "independence," "individuality," and "contract" tend to cluster together and with the idea of maleness or masculinity. These connections make up part of the "ideologies of the moral life" that are prominent in our culture, to borrow a phrase of Cheshire Calhoun's.[3] They are those ideas that form the horizon of moral imaginations, that incline us to look in certain directions for problems, solutions, and justifications, and nudge us to accept certain moral intuitions, analogies, and metaphors, without themselves pretending to be sound arguments for, or even good reasons to accept, any of these ideas (which is not, of course, to say that there may not be good reasons for promoting a certain ideology of the moral life, as well as good reasons for resisting others). The ways in which moral and political notions, images, and narrative threads have been bundled and gendered have significant effects on how we live and think publicly and communally, even if they may have only tenuous relationships with how particular individuals might experience and make sense of their own lives.

That these ideas have been so bundled and so gendered in our common imagination is in some sense an empirical claim, but one I take to be at least relatively uncontroversial: evidence is available from psychology,[4] intellectual and philosophical history[5], and from countless contacts with popular culture that are commonly experienced by people in contemporary America: when Garrison Keillor closes the "News from Lake Woebegone" with the tag line, "All the women are strong, all the men are good-looking, and all the children are above average," part of the humor resides in an inversion of standard gender associations; it is Ally McBeal, and not some male sitcom counterpart, who is haunted by a ghost baby. And so forth.

It has also been well established that notions that enjoy an association with the idea of maleness, if not necessarily with the subjectivities of actual men, have had a persistent edge in the competition for effective influence over cultural and political practice. When one turns to important political theorists such as Rawls, what one finds are images of rational self-interested individuals hammering out the terms of their lives together from their ignorance about themselves, not of compassionate agents acting out of their knowledge of each other. When one looks at the pecking order within academic disciplines such as philosophy or economics, what tends to be most prized is the most formal, the most abstract, the least connected with living everyday life, particularly as life is lived in familiar and intimate settings. And, particularly crucial for my purposes here, reigning moral and political theories strongly tend to start with an assumption that it is our distinctness, our separateness, that most faithfully signifies what is morally special about persons, and that it is those forms of human activity that broach the barriers between us that need special monitoring and justification.

But you needn't dismiss the importance of Rawls' views, the heuristic richness of formal methods, nor the moral significance of the separateness of selves to note that there is nothing necessary about either their associations with certain ideas of gender, nor with the way we allow those associations to make gratuitous additions to the cultural authority such ideas deserve on their own merits. In principle, we can both unbundle and reassociate these ideas, and in practice, we have no need to start from scratch as we do so. Ways of thinking about culture, philosophy, politics, and policy that are both carefully motivated argumentatively and which draw less on notions identified with the masculine are available to us—feminist approaches, most conspicuously, as well as some understandings of communitarianism—and these approaches may lead to justifying, and even installing, forms of practice that are more effective in responding to real needs. They may also help us clarify, and may resonate more deeply with, our best impulses. Insofar as they do, they themselves become more plausible as general pictures of what we should be most concerned about as we direct our own lives, and how we should live with one another. That they lack the imprimatur of a set of social practices that stubbornly continue to privilege what is associated with the masculine over what is associated with the feminine hardly counts as a reason to think otherwise.

ORGANS AS GIFTS

Yet before teasing out what might follow from looking at organ transplantation through the metaphor of pregnability, the claims of the current model need further consideration. The reigning attitude in the United States is that organs are not only items that we *may* regard as "gifts," but are, in fact, *essentially* gifts: we may freely withhold or freely give them, but we may not sell them, nor claim them from others as a matter of right, nor even regard the provision of organs as something that is a default assumption of how decent people living in a decent society will treat each other.

To think of human organs as gifts in this specially restricted way has the great merit of practically underscoring the notion that people are morally important in ways that go beyond how they may be resources for each other—the Kantian notion that persons have "dignity but not price" is reinforced here—as well as acknowledging the special relationship between persons and their bodies. The respect owed to persons is itself a scarce and precious resource: any kind of cavalier approach to that of which we are made might with some plausibility be seen as a threat to the coherence of moral attitudes that need protection and continuous renewal.

Yet, whatever its philosophical merits, the gift model has been disastrous for the growing number of people whose lives could be substantially extended via organ transplantation. According to the United Network for Organ Sharing, 4855 people died while on waiting lists for organs in 1998 alone; for the year ending 30 June 2001, the death total was up to 6043. The UNOS total for the years 1988–1998 is 32,449.[6] How many people might have lived longer had organs been available, but who never even made it to waiting lists, is unknown, as is the number of life-years that will be lost in the future, if current patterns prevail.

There has been a good deal of ingenuity and effort exerted within the gift model to try to close the lethal gap between generosity and need. U.S. states have "required request" laws, which mandate that family members be asked to donate organs from the bodies of relatives who have died under suitable conditions; driver's licenses include check-off boxes with which one can identify oneself as a donor; and images of cultural heroes, such as Michael Jordan, are employed to nudge people into being conscious of, and friendly to, the prospect of providing organs to others. Yet the gap continues to grow.

ALTERNATIVES: ARTIFACTS, ANIMALS, AND THE MARKET

With altruism seemingly stymied, there has been persistent interest in what is surely one of American society's strong suits—technological innovation. As enough transplant organs are not available as gifts, perhaps the solution is to build better artificial organs, or to unlock the intriguing potential of human stem cells to produce human organs, or to deepen our understanding of genetic engineering, so that human bodies can reliably employ retooled animal organs.

Thus far, however, these approaches have run into both technical disappointments and moral challenges of their own. The long story of the effort to create a totally implantable, permanently indwelling artificial heart, for example, is a cautionary tale of the labyrinthine complexities of both the biology of circulation and politics of technology; xenograft inspires increasing worries, not simply about the moral status of animals who might provide organs to humans, but about the potentially grave public health risks of crossing species barriers in this way.[7] Human embryonic stem cells, with their apparent ability to generate all types of human tissues, are intriguing, but at this point, little more. Further, the process of obtaining such cells, harvested as they are from the inner cell mass of human blastocysts, or from fetal gonadal tissue, is itself scarcely innocent of moral controversies.[8]

There seems no good reason, therefore, to think that human organs are going to be rendered technologically redundant any time soon. Consequentially, there has seemed to some to be growing reason to turn to America's other strong suit—the market. If conceptualizing organs as essentially gifts does not meet our needs, perhaps we should abandon that notion, and with it the idea that there is something morally objectionable about commodifying nonrenewable human body parts. If the law of supply and demand, as understood in free markets, were allowed to operate, then, so experience tends to indicate, supply will rise.

It would be unfair to think that unsettling the gift model in favor of seeing organs as saleable goods recommends itself solely to those who believe that the market is the fundamental form of moral relationship between people. Commodifying organs does not necessarily entail the prospect of people being surgically mutilated for profit during their life-times; that sort of transaction might well still be legally blocked, so long as enthusiasm for the market does not go so far as to welcome the prospect of impoverished people lining up to sell kidneys and liver lobes. What has been seriously suggested is a more modest, more pragmatic approach to enhancing organ availability through judicious application of mild economic incentives. We might, for example, test how supply is enhanced by providing families of recently deceased potential organ donors with various kinds of fiscal inducements, from defraying funeral or hospital expenses to straight cash payments. People might also be willing to sell "future interests" in their organs, receiving payments in return for a binding undertaking that their organs be used for transplantation, should they happen to die in circumstances that lend themselves to this purpose.

There are signs, then, that the social consensus that organs should be regarded as essentially being gifts is fraying. While the reluctance to turn objects so closely related to human beings as their nonrenewable organs into objects that take on a market value remains fairly robust, it faces a problem: by reserving human body parts from the market we underscore the special significance of the idea of a human being, but in so doing, we may in effect be endorsing the premature deaths of quite concrete instances of that class. This is precisely the paradox of the gift model: it underscores that moral significance of human beings, but fails to produce sufficient organs to meet a need whose deep seriousness is a function of that very significance itself! The market model promises to mobilize more transplantable organs, but encroaches on one of the most meaningful ways we have of proclaiming the special moral status of human beings: even in an era of the triumph of markets, humans retain a value that markets cannot calculate. This seems to be just the kind of situation that calls out for new ways of thinking, different models for understanding what is at stake.

PREGNABLE SELVES

Let's return, then, to the notion that organ transplantation creates a new way in which we can be responsible for each others' lives, a way that chips away at the picture of human beings as fundamentally discrete, separate selves, joining their lives intimately only rarely, and only with those they choose, or to whom they are related, as we say, "by blood." Organ transplant makes available a sense in which we are all potentially related to each other "by blood." We now all face the chance that we may be in a position to save another person's life by a method that crucially involves sharing our bodies with those we save.

Does this fact provide us with reason to think of sharing organs as a practice we should, in general, expect from each other? That failure to do so should not be regarded simply as a purely discretionary matter? That we have in fact a duty to provide organs useless to ourselves, but vital to others, unless we have special reason to withhold them?

Not independently of other premises, surely. However, such premises seem very much ready to hand. In fact, it might be maintained that there are arguments concerning our duties to provide needy others with organs not currently of any use to ourselves that are sufficiently strong as to render speculations about new ways of thinking about human selves and their relationships quite beside the point.

BENEFICENCE AND EASY RESCUES

The moral notion of beneficence is key to a simple, plausible argument for a presumptive duty to provide others with organs that may be vital to them but are useless to us. Beneficence is often characterized as the obligation to provide help to those in need, particularly in serious need, if the help can be rendered at little cost to the agent. Accepting such a duty seems to cohere closely, if not strictly follow from, the barest acknowledgment that people other than one's self (and those with whom one may have particular emotional ties) matter morally, and hence that their needs, interests, and projects have at least a presumptive moral value, too.

It's worth stressing just how minimal this assumption is. Accepting beneficence as a moral principle does not require accepting any substantial notion of impartiality, as utilitarianism tends to advocate; you needn't think that everyone's interests should count alike in your practical deliberations.[9] All that's required is to believe that other people's interests count for something that is not altogether negligible. Someone who dissented from this very weak form of beneficence, and yet who wanted to maintain that she did not regard other people as altogether bereft of moral worth, would presumably have to see the freedom to direct her own agency in whatever way she chose as having an extraordinary kind of super-value, one that comes within hailing distance of trumping all other moral reasons. Such a position is not without adherents, but it is, to put the matter gently, strongly counterintuitive.

Just how counterintuitive can be vividly appreciated by considering the "duty of easy rescue" most familiarly illustrated (and motivated) by stories about children tripping, hitting their heads, and falling stunned into shallow ponds. Confronted with such stories, most people will allow that not extracting from their predicament any such children as we might come across is gravely wrong, at least absent very strong reasons for acting otherwise. If personal freedom were a value strong enough to trump beneficence, then *any* contrary whim would be enough to exempt a non-rescuer from the charge of grave wrongdoing.

Easy rescue examples can be multiplied without strain, particularly if we are willing to settle for TV standards of fidelity to ordinary experience: one of those run-away trolley cars beloved of contemporary moral philosophers threatens to run over five people helplessly tied to the tracks, and, quite without inconvenience, you can push a switch diverting it to an unoccupied siding. Can individual liberty, worthy of reverence though it is, justify you in not pushing the switch?

But there's really no need to visit the philosophical trolley yard. There's nothing outlandish about imagining taking a stroll with someone absorbed in thought, who wanders into the path of an oncoming car. A sharp shout from you will effectively bring her to a more realistic grasp of her situation. Inaction in such cases may be in principle excusable, but as most will surely agree, you'd need to be supplied with unusually good reasons to avoid the conclusion that you had done something very wrong indeed if you kept your mouth shut. Freedom of the individual does not seem up to the job.

What can be learned from such examples? At least this, I think: there is a strong presumption that refusing to save another person's life, when doing so is virtually costless to the person in a position to act, is seriously wrong. And it might seem that the implications of this point for a duty to provide your organs to those in need, should it occur that you no longer have any need for them, are quite straightforward: absent some consideration that makes allowing one's organs to save the lives of other unusually burdensome, we all have a duty to take such steps as are readily available to bring it about that our organs are provided to others in need, should we happen to die in the appropriate ways.

Is this inference drawn too quickly? As I have already allowed, it is, for example, at least open to question whether organ transplantation is, all things considered, an appropriate way for societies to allocate their resources. Accordingly, so some might argue, any "duty to donate" might be defeated by considerations of justice. However, even if some system other than organ procurement and transplantation might be more efficient a method of making longer lives available to more people, it's not clear how that circumstance frees us from duties that confront us in the world as we find it. Building fences might be a more reliable way of keeping children from drowning in tempting ponds than is relying on the adventitious proximity of someone willing to get her sleeves wet. But the superior efficiency of fences hardly gives anyone good grounds not to rescue the child they happen to come across.

What does require extended attention is the idea that a person's relationship to parts of her body is not the same as her relationship to the things that she possesses, or, perhaps, even to the deeds she does. On the plausible notion that we do not so much own, but rather *are* our bodies, granting others the use of our organs, even if those organs no longer form parts of a living whole, is a matter of letting others have some of us. And once we realize this, or so someone might suppose, we will be less likely to think that the dire need of others underpins a beneficence, "easy rescue"–based duty such that the posthumous provision of organs is virtually costless, except to those with somewhat idiosyncratic values. Willingness to provide our organs to others after our own deaths can reasonably be seen as agreeing to a kind of intimacy that cannot be expected as a matter of a duty.

So the "easy rescue" argument may not be able to show on its own that a willingness to provide organs upon your death is a reasonable moral default assumption. It is precisely in response to this concern that the reason organ transplantation provides to reorient how we think of ourselves among others may turn out to be useful.

ORGAN DONATION AND/AS INTIMATE RELATIONSHIP

The idea that serving as an organ source involves a kind of intimate sharing of one's self is powerfully illustrated in Richard Selzer's short story, "Follow Your Heart."[10] The story revolves around a woman named Hannah, whose husband Samuel died three years earlier, on his thirty-third birthday, shot in the head while helping someone change a tire by the side of road. Hannah agreed that Samuel's organs should be harvested for transplant, and later receives a letter informing her that her "husband's liver has gone to a lady in McAlpine; the right kidney is functioning in Dallas; the left kidney was placed in a teenage girl in Galveston; the heart was given to a man just [her] husband's age in a little town near the Arkansas border; the lungs are in Fort Worth, and the corneas were used on two people right here in Houston . . ." (p. 52).

Hannah is not comforted by this letter. In fact, she starts to think of herself as suspended in limbo, not quite a wife, not quite a widow, her husband not alive, but not altogether dead. One night she dreams of her husband and another man, and watches as a surgeon extracts Samuel's heart and places it in the other man's chest, who then sits up, puts on his shirt, and goes on his way. On awakening, Hannah suddenly knows what she must do: "What was instantly made clear to her—it was so simple—was that she must go to find that man who was carrying Samuel's heart. If she could find him and listen once more to the heart, she would be healed" (p. 55).

And, of course, after overcoming many obstacles and much reluctance on the part of the recipient, one Mr. Pope, that is just what she does.

> Then Hannah bent her head and slowly lowered her ear toward his left, his secret sharing, nipple . . . Oh, it was Samuel's heart, all right. She knew it the minute she heard it. She could have picked it out of a thousand. Hadn't she listened to it just this way often enough? Hadn't she listened with her head on his chest, and heard it slow down after they had made love? It was like a little secret she knew about his body, and it had always made her smile to know the effect she had on him (p. 62).

The hour she spends listening to Samuel's heart in Mr. Pope's chest does indeed heal her. Selzer writes that she leaves with "the certainty that she had at last been retrieved from the shadows and set down once more upon the bright lip of her life" (p. 62).

"Follow Your Heart" explores organ transplantation as giving rise to a new set of meanings that are bound up with intimacy and renewal. The transplantation of Samuel's organs has changed his relationship to his wife in a way that his death alone would not; it has put her in a kind of intimate relationship with strangers that she otherwise would not have, and which she must acknowledge in an act of intimacy—an act that allows her life to go on, as her husband's postmortem intimacy with Mr. Pope allowed his life to go on. His story makes tolerably plain that there are dimensions to organ transplantation not quite captured by the easy rescue model.

Aaron Ridley has tried to turn an intuition like the one that seems to be driving Hannah into an argument. His target is the proposal that the dead should be seen as a source of organs for the needy living, without requiring anything in the way of explicit permission from an advance directive executed by the now-dead person, or even the consent of the family. This is not quite the same position being advocated here: it is possible that a person could have a duty to do something, while it is yet wrong for others to make her do it. But there is enough contact

between what Ridley wants to attack and I to defend to make a consideration of his view appropriate.

Although the dead are, Ridley allows, strictly speaking beyond
harm, to treat them as though they were on that basis simply resources
for the living is to misunderstand in a very general way just what
human beings are.[11] It is to see us as owning, rather than being, our
bodies. Ridley thinks that if we take the "no harm can come to the
dead" view as justifying routinely retrieving organs, then we have
accepted a justification that would allow any kind of use of dead bodies. He imagines using human organs as targets in a shooting gallery
set up to promote a charity, quite understandably refers to such a practice as "in appalling taste" and "vile," and intimates that the considerations that show why we properly respond to the shooting gallery
notion with repugnance shows, too, that routine harvesting of human
organs would also fail to acknowledge the respect appropriately due
to people.[12]

It is important that Ridley takes himself to be describing not just an
understanding one might reasonably have of the significance of one's
body, but a view that *must* be held, on pain of having otherwise a confused understanding of what human beings are and why they matter;
one gets the impression that he is concerned that any other view flirts
with a sort of dualism. However, there are a number of possible attitudes you can have toward your body without being confused, either
metaphysically or morally. You can reasonably think of the matter as
Ridley does: we are our bodies, dead or alive. Or, you might reasonably think that we are our living bodies, and when we die, we are no
longer to be identified with the nonliving body. On such a view, at
death we do not start existing as a corpse; we simply no longer exist.
Our corpse is a kind of property then, a part of the estate we leave
behind us.

There are no doubt other reasonable contenders. But a single alternative will do to counter Ridley's claim uniquely to accommodate our
intuitions regarding the shooting gallery scenario. Using parts of dead
human bodies as targets, even for charity, may be appalling because
human bodies deserve respect due to their tight correlations with living
human beings, and because to use them as targets is to use them as we
use cheap, disposable artifacts. If parts of human corpses are someone's property, this conclusion is not invalidated: flags, first editions,
and Flemish masterpieces are all property, and yet many people would
have a similar response if the Stars and Stripes, a Gutenberg Bible, or
Rembrandt's *Night Watch* were to be used for target practice. Further,

the kind of good that transplantation pursues is of deep moral significance and, generally, not available otherwise. Human organs are not
being used in roles for which we might as well as use paper bull's-
eyes or clay pigeons. Nor has transplantation the kinds of emotional or
symbolic resonance that the practice of plunging bullets into parts of
human bodies supports.

But rather than push these points further, I want to acknowledge the
power in Selzer's story, and to accept that a plausible way of accounting for that power is Ridley's contention that human organs are and
continue to be part of the human beings they originally helped to constitute. Would such an understanding provide a person with good reason to withhold her organs from someone who is likely to die if they
are withheld?

This, I think, depends on the general stance we take concerning the
relationship between ourselves and others, what we might call the
"default attitude." There are, as I have already suggested, powerful
cultural norms that install the attitude that our separateness is a greatly
important feature about human beings, taken to be closely connected
conceptually to integrity and dignity, and causally bolstered by its
association with masculinity as a culturally normative notion. Intimacy with others, in part because it imperils certain notions of normative masculinity, is seen as something of a threat to us, or at any rate
to many of us. But I do not believe that the only way we can acknowledge or cherish the significance of our distinctiveness or of our intimate relationships is by means of attitudes that have as a consequence
that thousands die what are in effect untimely deaths.

That we can give vital parts of ourselves to others, sustaining their
ability to act and to experience even after our own is gone, can be seen
as a highly concrete affirmation of our continuing interest, and indeed,
participation of a kind, in the weal of our communities after our own
deaths. The connection to pregnancy, and more broadly, to parenthood, is patent: if one of the ways in which people tend to see parenthood is as a way of continuing their own influence and interests into a
future they will not experience, and if part of what inclines us to see
the matter this way is our physical connection to our children, we
should be able to see organ transplantation in something of the same
way.

Indeed, this is not merely a way in which some people might come
to see organ donation—the next advertising strategy after "don't take
your organs to heaven with you" plays out. Rather, it's a construction
of the practice of organ sharing that we have strong moral reason to

accept, precisely since it avoids any cheapening of the significance of human beings, their parts, and their relationships, while extending human lives. I will now argue that the task of accepting this sort of view is not only a personal challenge, but a matter of public interest as well.

ORGAN PROCUREMENT AND POLITICAL PHILOSOPHY

I take it that "easy rescue"–type considerations provide us with strong presumptive reasons to provide organs for people who need them, even given an appropriate understanding of the significance of human organs and human intimacy; accepting Ridley's view of the relationship of human selves and human bodies does not derail this conclusion. We have available and should take seriously a way of thinking about ourselves and our relationships that endorses our metaphoric pregnability—that is, the ability of our bodies to sustain lives other than our own, and the affiliated notion that such an ability fosters moral attitudes that elevate connection over discreteness as the distinguishing way in which we think about ourselves as morally worthy beings. We have reason to accept such a view, because it is not inconsistent with any demonstrably correct understanding of who and what we are, and because it allows us to recognize and discharge duties of easy rescue, saving lives that other understandings squander.

Hence, I think that people typically have duties to provide organs to others, should the opportunity arise, and indeed, duties to reconsider and possibly to refigure their attitudes about themselves and others insofar as those attitudes threaten their inclinations to be organ providers. Or, to put it a bit more carefully, since it seems a bit strained to think of dead people having duties, I think that removing organs from the dead typically neither harms nor wrongs them, and that therefore we the living have a prima facie duty to support the retrieval of useful organs, both from our own dead bodies, and from those of others. If we find ourselves repulsed or otherwise distressed by this prospect, we have a derivative duty: to seek to revamp our attitudes.

It could be argued against this conclusion that the very need to revamp attitudes may make the duty in question no longer one of easy rescue, at least for many people; recalcitrant attitudes, difficult to shift, would not threaten simply our performance of our duty, but rather excuse us from it.

It is not immediately clear how serious this objection is. Ridley hoped to argue that seeing dead human bodies as a standing reserve of organs was inconsistent not simply with certain attitudes, but with attitudes backed by an appropriate understanding of what humans are and why they matter. But this view, I have argued, is mistaken; we can properly regard and honor ourselves while at the same time acknowledging the possibility and importance of the kind of intimate relationship with other people that transplantation involves, and the greater possibility of saving lives with such an attitude itself provides us with strong reason to endorse it. Imagine someone coming upon the drowning child who has a strong view about the importance of a carefully crafted appearance. She feels that her own dignity is importantly caught up with the way she and her surroundings look, and pays careful attention to maintaining the appearances. Pulling the child out of the pond can threaten the integrity of her look; rather than chic, she'll be soggy. Does this give her sufficient grounds to let the child drown?

This example has some analogies to the case at hand. Just as the feelings about the self Ridley describes are morally open to people, so there is nothing intrinsically wrong with the notion that human dignity can be effectively conveyed through careful attention to order and appearance; it is not as though the person's reluctance to rescue is a matter of prejudice against the ethnicity of the drowning child. But neither is the analogy perfect. The kind of individualistic understandings of self-and-body boundaries that drive the reluctance to donate organs being considered here are tolerably widespread and entrenched, more so, I'd be willing to admit, than the concerns about appearance of even the fastidious. What I think the analogy does show, however, is that our moral intuitions are not satisfied with an understanding of the easy rescue duty in which "easy" means roughly the same as "costless." More particularly, it suggests that, if we harbor attitudes that make otherwise easy rescues difficult, we have moral reason to wish things were different in our own psychic economies. In the light of easy rescue opportunities blocked by patterns of attitudes that seem themselves in some sense optional, such as a passion for order and style, we should desire that such attitudes would in the right circumstances be temporarily silenced. In the case at hand, we have reason to wish that a sense of violated boundaries might be transfigured into a more accommodating notion of ourselves and our relationships.

This consideration brings into play the social aspect of the question of organ retrieval, since social practices and understandings can do a great deal to install and nurture certain patterns of feeling. The question I now want to consider is whether we can regard providing organs to others as a practice that should form part of a collection of duties recognized socially, and facilitated through public policy and law. Could a good society enforce an organ provision duty, in a way at least weakly analogous to how conscription is enforced, or to take what is perhaps a better example, to how service on juries is mandatory? If a certain conception of human relationships facilitates that duty, may a good society foster it?

Proposing the details of a revised system of organ procurement is not part of my present ambition, but certain features of the policy I have in mind do need to be mentioned. I proposed a weak analogy between organ provision and such standing social duties as jury duty or the draft here in part because the standard for exemption from providing organs should, as I see it, be entirely subjective; if you want "conscientious objector" status, you can get it simply by self-proclamation. No review board nor judge need concur that your reasons are adequate, nor that you are sincere. So "opting out" would be an easy matter.

But it is important to be clear that a "presumed consent" policy is not what's on the table. The policy in question does not rest on the assumption that most people would consent to be organ donors. The animating principle, rather, is that, should the correct circumstances arise, people are obligated to provide organs unless excusing conditions are present, and that it is no abuse of state power to aid citizens in the exercise of this duty.

This last point might be thought to take some showing. In particular, it might be thought that justifying a communitarian understanding of the citizen–polity relationship would be required, particularly as I have suggested that fostering certain images of the nature and significance of human relatedness may well be a crucial role for the state to play. For it will surely strike many that liberal political philosophy will be inhospitable to such a role, or to a political recognition of this duty at all. Even if the moral arguments in support of a presumptive duty to provide organs were strong enough to do the job without the need for installing and promoting ideas about organ provision as opening up new possibilities for human intimacy, they should not be implemented politically. To do so would require relying on arguments drawing on specific, contestable understandings of the good. But that is precisely what liberalism abhors. This is true even if it could be shown that an understanding of beneficence strong enough to generate a duty to provide organs is very broadly recognized in a polity. The arguments purporting to show that there is a duty of beneficence are surely not so strong as to make a person flat-out irrational if she does not accept them. Further, if many of us would need to refashion our understanding of intimacy and of how to mark the significance of our bodies to remove barriers to appreciating the call of beneficence here, that would seem even more reason to expect a liberal political order to reject the notion that any such moral duty, involving not only a contestable notion of the good, but also the need to adopt new forms of self-understanding, could have political countenance.

Communitarianism, on the other hand, seems much more hospitable to recognizing a duty of organ provision. Communitarians don't, after all, have to worry about justificatory neutrality: if the value of providing organs is inseparable from some (set of) visions of the good, or if certain understandings of intimacy facilitate people's appreciation of the duty, that's not an in-principle problem. Cherishing the notion that people ought to see their own good as complexly intertwined with the good of others, and hence that we should do more for each other, might well be part of the conception of the good that a political community sees as part of its point to promote. Indeed, this might seem more than just a notional possibility: socially promoting beneficence seems to cohere with communitarianism's spirit, since communitarian theories of the self underscore the significance of "encumbrance," of identification with significant features of our communities, including its moral commitments, as an essential feature of a person's identity. A person's relationship to the community and its values is not, as it is on the liberal vision, ultimately a matter of choice exerted from some more or less noumenal perspective; the relationship between community and self-understanding, to what provides us with the "why" of our choices and actions, is much tighter— in part, at least, constitutive rather than elective.

If the analysis so far is on track, we're left with these questions: Is the ability to accommodate politically the conclusions for which powerful moral arguments can be made a mark in favor of a given political conception? If communitarianism is superior to liberalism in this respect, is that a reason to suppose it may be superior *tout court*?

It would seem that if tolerance is indeed as important a personal and political virtue as we generally assume (and as centuries of violence in the name of certain conceptions of the good would seem to demonstrate), then any such inferences would seem much too quick—or at least the operative sense of "reason to suppose" would have to be extremely weak. What would at least need to be shown to provide this political philosophy with any real support is that communitarianism—or, more precisely, some version of communitarianism—not only accommodates a significant moral conclusion that liberalism cannot, but that the form of communitarianism in question is no more likely to lead to disrespect, coercion, or violence toward dissenters than is its liberal rival.

The typical moves against liberalism include maintaining that its vaunted neutrality is overstated—that is, that its justificatory strategies are infused with certain contentious assumptions about what has value—while also maintaining that the kind of neutrality to which liberalism aspires in principle would render it practically ineffective if achieved. This has been well argued, to choose but one example, in Ezekiel Emanuel's *The Ends of Human Life*, where he focuses on medical ethical case studies to show that only specific, contestable constellations of values can put sufficient content into bioethical principles and policies for them to have a practical impact on deliberation and action.[13]

Such criticisms speak to whether liberalism, as a viable political philosophy, has a unique claim to tolerance and respect for value pluralism. If the criticisms are warranted, and liberalism is unable to function absent commitment to reasonably substantive, contestable values, then it becomes one political philosophy among others, not a referee for contending conceptions of the good, floating on a cloud of purely procedural justice far above the fray. Yet even seen as itself a conception of the good, it still has an important contribution to make to political life. We might reasonably assign it the job of vigilantly warning rival views about the dangers inherent in uncritically enacting policies that are justified by, and help entrench, richly contentful conceptions of the good, particularly (though not solely) on people who don't share those normative commitments. Such warning, however, along with appropriate responses, must proceed without pretending that public policy could altogether avoid drawing on such conceptions.

The liberal warning could be taken to heart by exposing policy proposals to various kinds of questions. One might be called the *convergence question*: is the moral goal in view, and the practices, virtues, and understandings that facilitate its attainment, reasonable from a variety of normative perspectives? Justifying a goal or practice simply by avowing, "this is our way," may make sense within certain communities, but it is not the best ground for putting the power of a modern state, embedded in a pluralistic culture, behind a policy. To the extent that a given policy suggestion can be motivated by a variety of viable moral and political perspectives, we have reason to suppose that enacting it won't wrong any of the polity's members.

A second query might be called the *fallibilism question*. A social policy that involves marshaling common resources in service of a certain conception of the good needs to strike a balance between a sincere endorsement of its characteristic constellation of values, and fallibilism—the recognition that the animating conception of the good could be mistaken in its views about what is most worth pursuing, or that the policy might be mistaken about how the good is best to be pursued. This goes beyond merely recognizing the durability of value pluralism. The point is not merely that, despite whatever a state might choose to do, not every inhabitant will accept the schedule of values reflected in its actions. Nor is it solely the moral conviction that respecting a person's conception of the good is caught up with respecting that person herself, important as such respect is. It is, rather, the epistemic point that, however good the considerations that speak in favor of a given ranking of goods, or in support of particular strategies for attaining them, it is possible that other considerations may come to show that this ranking or those strategies are mistaken. In honoring dissent, a community provides itself with an important resource for the continual renewal of its own moral visions.

A third concern might be called *least infringement*. It is surely reasonable to prefer those policies that expose dissenters to the least significant intrusions upon their way of life consistent with progress toward the goal.

In terms of these considerations, social policies designed to increase the availability of transplantable organs, and to foster a notion of human interrelationship that emphasizes what connects rather than what separates us, fare pretty well. There's clearly much more than "this is our way" to be said for the goal of increasing the availability of transplantable organs, and what there is to be said can be heard from a great many moral locations.

But what of the means to this end that have been suggested here? Is there not something more controversial in trying to get state backing for a particular vision of how people are related to one another? The answer to this sort of question depends, in part, on the extent to which one believes that neutrality about such matters is possible. Skeptics about neutrality—like myself—will think that modern states willy-nilly endorse and promulgate certain visions of human relationships. The issue is not, then, whether the state may do so, but rather, what are the appropriate constraints on which visions it chooses and which means it employs to install them? The same questions are pertinent for means as for ends: to the extent that the means are reasonable, in that they do not impose heavy burdens on dissenters, and that dissent is both possible and honored—in that, for example, the means are promulgated in ways that do not bypass rational agency and are themselves open for review and debate—the view should pass muster.

How might government power facilitate a wider appreciation of other ways of looking at human relationships? In large part, such shifts require much in the way of cultural, rather than political, support, and "mediating structures" would no doubt have a good bit to do in reorienting the way people think about themselves and others. Organ procurement might well serve as a useful lever for unsettling normative views of human relationships now current. Imagine, for example, religious leaders discussing organ procurement in terms that stress duty and relationship, rather than gift and discretion, or imaginative writers and other artists exploring the pregnability metaphor. But the very movement by government authorities toward what would in practice amount to an "opt-out" system—including the political debates that would no doubt occur—would make available the thought that there are alternatives to understanding others' uses of one's organs as a gift, and that, although those alternatives require specific conceptions of the good and of the significance of human relationship, such conceptions have much to be said for them.

Reasonable forms of communitarianism—those that appreciate the epistemic and moral consequences of pluralism—have this advantage over prevailing understandings of liberalism, I believe: they allow for, and even encourage the possibility of, political discourse about ends, and not just means, about the kind of people we should be, and the kind of communities in which we should live. It seems to me possible to engage in such discourse, and even to come to certain practical conclusions as a result of deliberation, that are not essentially oppressive or alienating; indeed, quite the contrary. If organ provision and similar easy rescues are to be acknowledged as defeasible civic duties in U.S. public policy, we will need to reflect about what kind of people we are, what kind of people we want to be, and how we might move, both individually and as a community, from here to there. Neither pluralism nor fallibilism entails that large-scale polities are either morally or practically barred from discussing ends, and from using commodious conceptions of the good, emerging from appropriately structured forms of reasoning, as the basis of social policy, so long as appropriate provisions for dissenters are in place.

And finally, while I don't regard seeing the provision of organs as a duty rather than as a choice as inherently illiberal (easy rescue arguments, with ample accommodation for dissenters, probably are justifiable in the kinds of liberal polities that allow any form of presumptively mandatory contribution, such as service on juries, to the community), it seems to me that it is more likely to be a part of the social policy of a country that considers connectedness, or as it is more ordinarily called, solidarity, as a social value along with liberty, and can engage in political discussion about how such goods relate to each other. In fact, organ procurement policy as an expression of solidarity does not merely facilitate the recognition that postmortem provision of organs falls under the scope of easy rescue duties, but constitutes the basis of an argument for the duty to provide which is motivationally and conceptually distinct from easy rescue, lacking the calculations of benefit to others versus harms to self that easy rescue suggests. Given communitarian understandings of the relationship between people and the groups in which they live, understanding organ procurement through the lens of the pregnability metaphor can turn the availability of these life-extending resources from a "convergent" to a "common" good, to use a distinction of Charles Taylor's—that is, from something we all happen to value from the perspective of its contribution to our own ends, to something we value because it represents our acknowledgment of each other's worth.[14] Taylor has argued, persuasively in my view, that the availability of common goods actually enhances rather than threatens the legitimacy of political orders.

Many individual fates have been touched by organ transplantation, and many more might be. But there are other benefits lying latent in this nexus of technology and social practices, benefits not just to individuals, but to communities: a deepened appreciation of our interdependence, desire for common weal, and not only individual prospering. Ironically, to obtain a richer helping of the individual benefits, we may need to think more creatively about a topic that high-tech medical innovation is not much associated with, in fact has often been presented as inimical to—the fate we share as beings both mortal and social.

NOTES

1. Guido Calabresi and Philip Bobbit, *Tragic Choices* (New York: W. W. Norton, 1978).

2. Carol Gilligan, *In a Different Voice* (Cambridge, Mass.: Harvard University Press, 1982).

3. Cheshire Calhoun, "Justice, Care, Gender Bias," *Journal of Philosophy* 85 (1989): 451–63.

4. See Gilligan, *In a Different Voice.*

5. See Elizabeth Lloyd, *The Man of Reason: "Male" and "Female" in Western Philosophy* (New York: Routledge, 1993).

6. UNOS OPTN Scientific Registry Data, current as of February 1999, available at www.unos.org. The 2001 data is from the Scientific Registry of Transplant Recipients website at ustransplant.org, administered by the University Renal Research and Educational Association in collaboration with the University of Michigan (accessed 18 April 2002).

7. Laura Purdy and Peter Collingnon, "Xenografts: Are the Risks So Great that We Should not Proceed?" *Microbes and Infection* 3/4 (2001): 179–83.

8. James Lindemann Nelson, "Ethics and Embryos," *Forum for Applied Research and Public Policy* 15, no. 1 (spring 2000): 49–53.

9. See, for example, James Rachels, *The Elements of Moral Philosophy*, 3rd ed. (New York: McGraw-Hill, 2000), 115.

10. Richard Selzer, "Follow Your Heart," *Redbook*, September 1990.

11. For reasons I will not go into here, I don't agree that the dead are beyond all harm. I do think that the dead are not generally any the worse off simply for the removal of organs.

12. Aaron Ridley, *Beginning Bioethics* (New York: St. Martin's Press, 1998), 257–58.

13. Ezekiel Emanuel, *The Ends of Human Life* (Cambridge, Mass.: Harvard University Press, 1991).

14. Charles Taylor, "Cross-Purposes: The Liberal-Communitarian Debate," in *Liberalism and the Moral Life*, ed. Nancy L. Rosenbaum (Cambridge, Mass.: Harvard University Press, 1989).

7

Cloning, Families, and the Reproduction of Persons

The reproduction of human persons may be biologically exhausting, but it is not exhaustively biological. Nurturing our young, forming and consolidating their personal identities and interpersonal roles, and helping them become sensitive to the reasons the world presents to them for entertaining certain thoughts, and engaging in certain actions, are reproduction's social tasks, continuing the process initiated in conception, gestation, and parturition. People have proven extremely resourceful in developing different practices and structures for discharging these jobs and have understood what constitutes their successful completion in different ways. But all these strategies converge on assigning very important roles to small-scale intergenerational associations of people in which special forms of interpersonal acknowledgment and recognition go on. I refer, of course, to families.[1]

People have also shown themselves to be most ingenious in coming up with different approaches to the biological side of the reproduction of persons, the prospect of human reproductive cloning being a particularly conspicuous example of this ingenuity. Juxtaposing these social and technological reproductive strategies introduces the general question I want to consider in this chapter: if cloning were to be added to the array of options for carrying out the biological aspects of human reproduction, how might the remaining tasks involved in reproducing persons, as they are embedded in family structures familiar to many of us, be affected? I'll be emphasizing ways in which those social tasks might be rendered harder to complete well, might become less certain of their ends, or might be more likely to be frustrated—that is, the possible negative implications that cloning human beings might have for families.

This might seem like so much abuse of what is clearly already a corpse of an issue; while therapeutic cloning has serious advocates and a serious point, the enthusiasts for using cloning to make children, rather than stem cells, all seem to have rather curious motives—consider, for example, the Raelians, a sect of UFO enthusiasts whose members see cloning as a move toward personal immortality. With advocates like that, does reproductive cloning really need critics?

Yet what is now firmly on the other side of the pale is not guaranteed to stay put. In my view, the most familiar arguments are far from water-tight; repugnance is playing a large role in the social and political rejection of reproductive cloning, and it's too early to say whether that repugnance emerges from wisdom or folly, or whether it will endure. As it happens, I don't regard the arguments I'll offer here as knockdown, drag-out demolitions of cloning either. Rather, they highlight threats cloning poses to families, threats that certain understandings of cloning, and attendant policies, might avoid—but not, of course, unless those dangers are first noticed.

I also will stay alert to ways in which human reproductive cloning might actually facilitate a family's efforts to achieve important parts of its social reproductive tasks, parts connected with contributing to the world's becoming a more just place. So this chapter might have been called "Two Boos for Reproductive Cloning." In the present context, that almost amounts to half a cheer.

CLONING PERSONS: SOME MOTIVATIONS

I'm not tempted by the view that cloning *as such* is a threat to families, or to anything else of value; my approach is to situate this technology within various motives for its employment, and try to make out what may emerge from different constellations of hopes for its use. So I'll start by roughing out some more-or-less generalizable situations or "scenarios" in which cloning might seem an attractive reproductive option; this does not pretend to be a complete catalog but will include a number of the motivations that have been most widely discussed. The first scenario I will call *exclusion*: a person might wish to have a child that lacked a specific kind of genetic link that, but for cloning, would be present. A woman who carried the gene that causes Huntington disease, for example, might want to bear a child who is genetically related to her husband, and not (except for mitochondria) to her.

Screening fertilized ova prior to implantation and discarding those with the Huntington gene presents her with an alternative to cloning, but if she sees discarding preembryos as tantamount to abortion, it may be an option she cannot elect. Such a woman would still achieve her goal by having the nucleus of one of her husband's cells inserted into her enucleated egg and then bringing the resultant fetus to term.

But genes can be problematic for reasons other than the proteins they code for; there's a more directly social dimension to exclusion, too. Consider a lesbian couple that wants to have a child who is genetically related to one partner and gestationally to the other, but not genetically related to any male parent. For such a couple, cloning seems just the ticket: a cell nucleus from one partner and an enucleated ovum from the other permits the partners, but no one else, to be the most proximate biological cause of their child's existence.

Next, I'll consider a scenario I call *replication*. A straightforward example: a couple shares a wish to reproduce via cloning in order to replace a deceased child as closely as possible, imagining that their dead child's appearance and personality will strongly tend to recur in the cloned child. But "cloning-for-replication" could be even more attractive as a technique to forestall a child's death.

Mary Ayala and her husband Abraham acted out of this sort of motive in bringing their daughter Marissa-Eve into the world in April of 1990. The Ayalas had thought themselves quite done with expanding their family—in fact, Mr. Ayala had been sterilized—when their sixteen-year-old daughter Anissa was diagnosed with chronic myelogenous leukemia. She needed a bone marrow transplant from someone with whom she was histologically compatible, but strenuous searching revealed no suitable donor. So, the Ayalas tried to make one.

They had a lot of hurdles to clear. Mr. Ayala had to have a vasectomy of seventeen years' standing effectively reversed, Ms. Ayala had to become pregnant at forty-two, the child had to be a compatible donor for her sister (only a one in four chance there) and, even with a bone marrow transplant, Anissa had no guarantee of achieving a long-term remission.

The Ayalas beat all those odds.[2] But if a use of cloning that straddles the "reproductive-vs.-therapeutic" distinction had been available, they wouldn't have had to face at least some of them. If Anissa had been cloned, her father's sterilization would not have been an issue. Nor would her mother necessarily have been the person to gestate the fetus. Most dramatically, the incompatibility concerns would not have arisen—Anissa would have been assured of a match as perfect as possible.

Circumstances of this sort make reproductive cloning for organ and tissue transplantation a very intriguing option. So attractive an option, perhaps, that some couples would be interested in cloning ova fertilized *ex utero* as a more-or-less routine matter, cryropreserving one of the embryos as insurance against the day when its tissues—or possibly even its organs—might be crucial to the welfare of its born twin.

A third kind of interest in cloning revolves around what I will call *affirmation*. Here, the aim is to employ reproductive cloning to mark a relationship in some special fashion. Imagine a woman mourning the death of a much-loved partner. No gametes from that partner are available, but viable somatic cells are, and she wishes to bear a child in her partner's image as a living testimony to their love. Or perhaps she uses nuclear material from a child they have already had together, with the same motivation—not to replace the child, but to express an ongoing commitment to the father. A variation on this theme has been suggested by William Ruddick, who imagines a husband so smitten by his wife that he wants to have the experience of raising someone as much as possible like her when she was young.[3]

These motivations are not, of course, mutually exclusive. Some lesbians, for example, might be motivated as much or more by a desire to express their mutual love and commitment, than by the desire to exclude from their reproductive lives any elements they find undesirable there. At the same time, there are significant distinctions among the scenarios, a feature that complicates any moral discussion of human reproductive cloning per se. Yet there is a feature that runs through all of them: the marked importance they place on biological relationships. Getting a decent purchase on the moral implications of reproductive cloning will, I believe, require trying to better understand why such relationships are so significant to so many of us.

THE MEANINGS OF BIOLOGICAL CONNECTEDNESS

The significance of genetic near-indistinguishability is perhaps most straightforward in "Ayala"-type cases, in which a new child is desired, at least in large part, for the medical benefits her body offers to another family member.But even where matching body parts aren't the issue, we find that in each scenario—the lesbian couple who thinks it important for both of them, and only them, to be involved in their child's coming into the world, the grieving couple who wishes to retain as strong as possible a link to their lost child, the widow who wishes to keep alive her connection to her husband—it's a biological idiom that is seen as having the most power to express the various exclusions, replications, and affirmations.

There is nothing out of the ordinary about the significance many people place on biological ties. The most telling, ubiquitous instance is the common and profound interest in reproducing children: most people are not indifferent between the reproductive options of having children "of their bodies," so to speak, and adoption. The cause of this common preference is, no doubt, overdetermined: the sociobiologists have an explanation,[4] and, on top of the considerations they advance, it is for many people simply much easier to beget and bear than to adopt, and it may strike them too as a more reliable way of getting children who can be counted on not to present their parents with unpleasant surprises. But I can't bring myself to think that these considerations fully explain the depth or the prevalence of this desire. For one thing, having children of one's own body is *not* always easier than adoption—consider what some people, especially women, go through by way of assisted reproduction. Nor is it always all that reliable a way to steer clear of surprises, as experienced parents know.

I'm inclined to think that another important part of many people's interest in having "their own" children is a response to their sense of their mortality, but also, more generally, to their temporality, to being creatures whose births, lives, and deaths take place within a brief part of a very long stretch of time.[5] Bringing new children into the world can be both a powerful expression of interest in the future and a way of connecting ourselves to what will transpire long after we're no longer on the scene. Nor is the past irrelevant. The history many people share of being children cared for by parents can lend to the prospect of being parents caring for children a sense of deep coherence with some of the most basic rhythms of our form of life. Too, begetting, bearing, and rearing children is a way of participating in, and pushing further, the ongoing stories of the particular families in which we live.

Clearly, these are not the only reasons why most people prefer to have children of their own bodies, and for some they may not even be part of the reason. If the connection to the future motif were a uniquely and universally powerful motive for reproduction, cloning would seem an extraordinarily attractive strategy, not an emotionally repugnant one. What cloning conspicuously lacks, as least for heterosexual people, is the biologically mediated mingling of lives, histories, and futures afforded by sexual reproduction. That kind of joining may help explain why many people interested in having children are also interested in having them with particular other adults—surely, a more widely distributed motivation than is an indifference about the person with whom one has children, as long as one can decide with whom one will raise children.

So I'm not suggesting that these ideas fully explain why biological connections to our children seem so compelling a part of these pictures. If we hope that something important will testify to our having been a part of the world once we've left it, why would not enduring social achievements serve as well? Because it's harder to write a memorable novel than to give birth to a child and raise her well? If we want to underscore our place in a particular historical framework, evidence of continuity is all around us, as close as the language we speak. And many people have found raising adopted children deeply satisfying. Is the general interest in whose gametes are involved in a child's being in the picture in the first place just a result of ignorance of the joys of adoption?

My tendency is to think that our interest in biological reproduction has something important to do with the fact that our biological children strike many of us as our fullest and most faithful representatives as particular, embodied persons. We have something in common with children we have conceived, born, or begotten that we cannot have with nonrelatives, no matter how thoroughly we may have shared our lives with them. This is of course just a speculation in what is basically an empirical matter, but it is not essential to the points I am trying to bring out that I be correct about it. In fact, it is interesting that my speculations about why biology matters so much to so many—like other such speculations of which I am aware—seem to fall short of fully coming to grips with the reality of what they're trying to explain. That suggests that whatever the truth about the meaning of biological connection happens to be, it is complex, varied, overdetermined, and deep.

What is important is that we accept that biological considerations are very significant to many people. Some observers have suggested that our special engagement with our kin is a socially constructed matter, and I have no particular quarrel with that unless branding something as a social construct implies that it is fundamentally unimportant, ontologically second-rate, and practically an easy matter to shift. There need be nothing whimsical or second-rate about our interest in biological connectedness with other persons, however that interest is installed.

That acknowledged, however, we must also be clear that biological connections do not trump all other sources of importance. Nor does whatever interest we may have in extending those connections deserve to be encouraged, whatever direction it may happen to take. We may easily misinterpret or misdirect or otherwise misunderstand the importance of our biological affiliations. Indeed, the worries I have about cloning and families are prompted by two such concerns. First, biological connectedness may matter to children, not just to adults. Second, it is possible to assign too much significance to biological connectedness.

Let's start with the first of these points—biological connections matter to many children as much as they do to many parents. Consider those children raised by loving and competent adoptive parents, who yet retain an interest in knowing who their genetic parents are and in seeking out some kind of relationship with them. Some children whose conception was effected through artificial insemination by a donor (AID) have expressed similar interests, reporting that the lack of knowledge about, and lack of relationship with, their progenitors is very painful.[6] Both adoption and AID traditionally have been arranged in ways that slight children's interest in knowing their biological parents. But this is at least somewhat curious, surely, in a society willing to go to such lengths to bring about biological connection between adults and the children they raise. Why should we so privilege adult interests and so dismiss the interests of children? Why, to put the question in terms of my speculation about the matter, should we regard a biological connection to the future as a vital part of the identity of adults, but not see biological connectedness to the past as an equally vital part of the identity of children?

BIOLOGICAL MEANINGS, SOCIAL CONSTRUCTIONS, AND THE EXCLUSION SCENARIO

Children's interest in biological connection is not a problem for all motivations for reproducing persons via cloning, but it does make a bit of trouble for some of them. Consider the variation of the exclusion scenario that involves lesbian parenthood. Would this use of cloning present any creditable threat to the successful completion of the nonbiological tasks involved in the reproduction of persons? Possibly, in a world such as ours, "radical fatherlessness" might be distressing to some children. If we think of children brought into the world in this way as "genetically single-parent children," then if they had any desire analogous to that reported by some children conceived via AID—to know the absent male biological parent—the circumstances of their birth would seem to render it a perfectly useless passion.

I do not disregard the importance of such "fatherlessness feelings" as there may be, but this is not actually the consequence I find most troubling. While it is not implausible to think that some children may feel some distress at this feature of their lives, I do not know whether it is plausible to expect many to be altogether devastated by such news. Further, *just those children* could not have been born in any other fashion than cloning, so any objections to not having a father would seem to be objections to conditions essential to their own lives.

What concerns me more is that this kind of exclusion rests not just on the technology of cloning, but upon what is, in effect, a social decision to maintain what might be called the "moral distinctness" of generations. But is that decision self-evidently the right one? Will the child herself necessarily agree that her mothers have been successful in blocking genetic connectedness to a male parent and that therefore she has no father? The child is, after all, very largely genetically identical to the person who contributed the nucleic material for the cloning procedure, a person who was herself conceived in the usual way. Suppose that the father of the nucleus contributor is alive. If so, the child born via cloning is genetically almost indistinguishable from his child. If the cloned child is on the lookout for a father, this man might seem to be a good candidate.

Indeed, rather than see this child as a "genetically single-parent child," we might see her as having *three* genetic parents—the nucleus donor and both of *her* parents—and a gestational/mitochondrial parent. Or perhaps the best way to put it is that the child has a gestational mom, a genetic mom and dad, and a sister who happens to be an identical twin despite being, say, a quarter of a century older, and the gestational mom's spouse as well.

I do not believe that there is any good argument showing that such an arrangement should seem "appalling to all people of good moral judgment" or anything of that kind. There is no reason in principle why we could not relax and refigure prevalent notions of the moral distinctness of generations and of familial and gender roles more generally. Indeed, in some respects we *should* do so, and in some respects this is done. While the patterns of moral understandings most heavily represented in the United States today customarily freight the roles of parent, grandparent, and sibling with very different kinds of expectations and obligations, there are surely times when these roles do overlap, quite without any intervention by cloning.[7] But here's the rub: who will have authority to determine what the relationships are in families of this sort—who is sister, who is mother, who is father, who is grandparent—particularly if the maturing child does not like the definitions she is handed?

What makes this situation potentially a tough one is the fact that decent cases can be made out both for the position of the putative child, who wants to ladle on her mother's father a kind of relationship that is heavily encumbered with significant duties—the role of being *her* father—and for the position of that man, who may have not the slightest interest in having anything to do with the child at all. Complicating things still further is that the decent cases I can imagine here rely on rather distinct kinds of moral understandings. The man can rely on a widely cherished principle in liberal political theory, the "no positive obligations without consent" principle. In other words, he can point out that he never agreed in any sense, expressly or tacitly, to be this child's father or anything in the neighborhood thereof, and plausibly be thought to have made a telling moral point. The child can reply that families are precisely the place where such a principle limps badly—traditional ideas of children's duties to their parents owe nothing to any such consent principle, for example—and rely for her part on the moral notion that people have special obligations to those who are specially vulnerable to them, particularly if they have been involved in the creation of the relevant vulnerability.[8]

The man in such a case might find himself in a position not dissimilar to a responsible truck driver who, through no fault of her own, has just struck someone darting out from between parked cars.Such a driver is ex hypothesi not negligent, and she certainly did not choose to go out and run someone over. At the same time, she should neither feel the same nor act the same about the accident as someone merely reading about it over her cereal the next morning.[9]

I focus on this sort of case because facilitating parenthood for homosexual people strikes me as one of the ways in which cloning could make a positive contribution to our social lives. If part of what we must do in raising children is to make them sensitive to patterns of injustice and to encourage them to resist oppression, we should support practices that may allow lesbians to enjoy a fuller range of the

goods of reproduction. But in a circumstance like this, human reproductive cloning seems prone to propel us into a situation in which we
face something of an antinomy. Children born of such arrangements
may have claims against the parents of the person who supplies the
nucleus, claims whose honoring may be important to a child's developing sense of her place in the narrative of her family, relating to her
sense of rootedness in the world—her particular place in its history. I
am concerned that these claims will not be heard, or, having heard
them, that we will not know how to honor them well—particularly as
they collide with other, morally well-founded claims that center on the
importance of autonomy in the lives of persons, on the importance of
not being "drafted" without consent into burdensome and prolonged
duties.

THE AFFIRMATION SCENARIO

A man learns that he suffers from a terminal illness. He and his wife
both find comfort in the idea of conceiving a child together before he
dies, and they do so, in the time-honored fashion. Should this cause us
to raise a moral eyebrow? Would the social side of reproduction be
unlikely to go well for this child? Would matters be any different if the
man were unable to reproduce sexually, but could supply healthy
somatic cells for reproductive cloning?

There may be some ground for concern even if the couple can avail
themselves of the "natural" method. Raising a child by oneself is a
tough job, and one cannot help but wonder a bit about the expectations
that the child will have to face. But we hardly seem likely to develop
a social policy forbidding such decisions. Would the resultant child's
circumstances differ importantly from those of a child brought into the
world via cloning for a similar reason?

The paradigm case here involves individual adults acting alone to
conceive a child; cloning is, of course, a case of assisted reproduction,
involving the agency of other people. How much should that matter?
Should assisted reproduction generally be thought of according to an
adoption model, in which candidates for parenthood have to satisfy
certain criteria to be given the charge of children—criteria that would
presumably exclude the imminent demise of one of the prospective
parents? Or should assisted reproduction generally be thought of as an
extension of the agency of the principals, the involvement of other

people being as morally "transparent" as is the involvement of a mid-wife at a normal birth?

A significant disanalogy between adoption and other forms of becoming a parent seems plain: in adoption, and not in biological reproduction, assisted or otherwise, someone (the "natural" parent, the adoption agency) is already responsible for an existing child, and must determine whether their relinquishment of that responsibility to another is a morally defensible act. Still, people involved in assisted reproduction are not quite in the same position as an obstetrician or a midwife assisting at a birth; irrefutable evidence of confirmed child abuse would not be relevant to aiding a delivery, but it does seem relevant to retrieving ova for in-vitro fertilization.

The question about whether it is appropriate for adults to reproduce in circumstances in which they would probably not be allowed to adopt assumed some prominence early in 2002, when a thirty-year-old woman with the genes for an unusual form of early onset Alzheimer Disease used preimplantation genetic diagnosis to have a child who would not be born with the same genetic abnormality that will almost certainly affect her mother within the next several years.[10] Bioethicists commenting on the *JAMA* article reporting this case offered an approach ostensibly not dissimilar to the one taken here: they worried about the impact on the social tasks of reproduction of a technology that allowed a woman with a very short life expectancy to bring a child into the world, and argued that resolving the matter of whether such a technology ought to be used in such a case hinged on whether reproduction was "a mere want, a deeply held desire, or a need so profound and fundamental as to trump the rights or needs of others."[11] For these writers, the answer to this question determines the status of reproduction in general. Is having children merely a privilege, or is it an "unquestionable and unalienable right"?[12]

Of course, reproduction, either with or without benefit of high-tech assistance, could be *neither*—neither a mere privilege (who is in a position to confer it?), nor an absolute right (could it really trump every countervailing consideration?). It might be more plausibly seen as an interest with respect to which adults have a serious but not irrebuttable presumption to be allowed to satisfy—at least, if they can arrange the willing cooperation of those others who may be needed for the enterprise to succeed. But even were the interest in reproduction either a right or a privilege, it could still be asked whether the people involved were discharging their privilege or their right in a responsible way. Does having a child in a situation in which it is likely that she will lose a parent early constitute irresponsibility? With that thin a description, it is impossible to tell; there may be a network of rich and resilient support awaiting the child. Yet the description seems thick enough at least to place just that question squarely on the table. Will the child reliably be provided with the relationships and resources she needs to have a reasonable chance to flourish? Will the child run a serious risk of having to make do with less than she has a reasonable claim to?

I have already suggested that, although children born as clones might not have any reasonable claim that their very existence wrongs them, they might well have a claim, which we are not well prepared to evaluate, to forms of relationships that we are not well-equipped to supply.

But in the kind of case I'm thinking about now, all of these problems can be largely stipulated away. Suppose the husband—or the woman in the previous scenario, for that matter—had no living parents or had parents willing to be significantly involved in the baby's life. Conflicts about identities and role would be less likely to emerge. Note, too, that cloning in the case that opens this section might be seen to be almost incidental or, at most, instrumental. The real point is just to have another baby together. Cloning may be attractive because it is the only way of doing so.

And yet, I worry still. For one thing, it might be difficult, as a matter of practice, to distinguish between couples taking a purely "instrumental" view of cloning (the point is to have a child, and as it turns out, cloning is all that will serve), and people who are drawn by the idea that cloning will give them a child that is specially suited to the purpose of affirming a relationship precisely because of its striking similarities to the deceased (someone who thinks of the child as "my husband returned," or something of the kind.) The second concern is that it might be difficult to sort out the matter even within ourselves. As I have noted, biological connection can have strong powers over our actions and imaginations, and strong physical and temperamental similarities between children and much-loved departed spouses might make the task of contributing to the development of the child's sense of his own, distinct, personal identity even more difficult than usual.[13]

If the problem we faced in the exclusion scenario was the risk of not taking children's interests in genetic connections seriously enough, the problem we face here is in taking the parents' interests in genetic connections so seriously as to lessen the chances that a child's interests in individuation would be well served. The reply is surely open that this

is more mere speculation, and, with some reservations about that qual-
ifying "mere," it's hard to deny this. The problem, I think, has a
sharper edge to it in connection with "replication" scenarios, which I
will discuss next. But before proceeding there, I want to try to forestall
one kind of misunderstanding. It would not be a good reply to this
concern to point out that "cloning is the only way *that* child could
have gotten here, and it's not likely that his interests in individuation
are going to be so pronounced, or so violated, that his life will be
worse that never having been born." The lessened chance of successful individuation that is our concern here is *not* a necessary consequence of its being in the world at all. A child born of cloning could,
at least in principle, at least for all we know, develop a robust and
secure sense of herself as an individual. Rather, the problem is that
there is reason to believe that parents who see their offspring's status
as a clone as key to its desirability in their family, might be particularly poorly placed to help the cloned child meet that need, thus violating her ongoing claim to establish a firm sense of herself.

THE REPLICATION SCENARIO

Being drawn to cloning as a reproductive means is often associated in
the popular mind with something like replacement: we desire to reproduce via cloning largely because our cloned child is thought to replicate some other individual, not because cloning is a means to
reproduction otherwise blocked or problematic. We fondly imagine
another child just like our lost David, another child with bone marrow
just like our desperately ill Marie's, even another dancer just like Baryshnikov.

If families' social reproductive tasks include the formation of identity, and if that job involves providing children with both the means to
identify with others and to individuate from them, it does not take too
much imagination to foresee some added difficulties here.[14] Achieving
the right balance between attachment and separation is hard enough
under the very best of circumstances. Imagine the fears that might
haunt people who had to accept that among the hopes cherished by
those responsible for their birth is the expectation that they would fulfill not just a certain role—not just take the preordained place in the
family business—but replicate a certain identity. With regard to at
least this motivation for reproductive cloning, it looks as though the
means and the morals are pretty much directly at odds, that the pro-

spective parents who turn to this technique are setting themselves up to fail at one of the trickiest and more important tasks of responsible reproduction.

Nor is putative psychological stress the only problem that cloned kids are going to have to face in their effort to establish themselves. No one is going to dance like Baryshnikov unless he works like Baryshnikov, and perhaps not even then. Suppose David showed an early flair for finance, and was remarkably successful in investing his lawn-mowing money in stocks; if David$_2$ lacks any such interest or aptitude, is he going to have to feign one? What if the market is just off during his youth? If, as I have assumed throughout, the reproduction of persons is not solely biological but also social, then effective "replication cloning" may require degrees of compulsory training or other kinds of character formation that go beyond what children require for basic socialization. Joel Feinberg has plausibly argued that children have some moral claim to kinds of education that leave them with a tolerably "open future"; getting what adults look for out of replication cloning threatens to restrict their futures in worrisome ways.[15]

Again, it might be rejoined that the situation these children will face is, while perhaps not optimal, not devastating either. Lots of children are kept hard at work at the barre for hours more than they would like and do not necessarily feel inclined to end it all rather than go on. Why think things would be worse for the young Mikhail? David$_2$ may resent having been pressured by his parents to put the whole of his paper route's annual proceeds into blue chips, but he may of course weather such resentment well—kids seem fairly resilient about such matters—and this resiliency may be shared even by desperately ill Marie's younger twin, who has to deal with the fact that she was brought into the world expressly to serve as a tissue or organ donor for her sibling. The "Ayala variation" does of course highlight the problem of whether such a child is being seen as a means to an end solely, but that is a highly contestable matter and clearly not strictly a matter of cloning. It may well be that the dignity accorded to any child is not a matter determined by the motivations that propelled her into existence, but by the way she is treated once she is among us; disrespectful treatment, unfortunately, is a risk all children face.[16]

But it seems to me that the moral issue here is not settled simply by adverting to the possibility that a cloned child may be loved for herself alone and not just for her yellow hair—or her bone marrow—nor by pointing out that lots of children born in ways wholly innocent of technology have tough childhoods and face real challenges in the way of successfully consolidating their identities. The issue involves, rather, identifying clearly and vividly how cloning might heighten risks, as well as offer benefits, and keeping clear who are the potential recipients of the harms and benefits, who are the responsible agents, and what are the live alternatives.

BEYOND "SMOKING GUN" BIOETHICS: CLONING, FAMILIES, AND PRUDENCE

In looking at the ways in which cloning might complicate the jobs families undertake in completing the reproduction of persons, I have found a good deal that troubles me, but nothing that quite counts as an ethical smoking gun—no evident and inescapable violation of accepted rights, no unambiguous and grave harm inevitably attached to human cloning under any of the scenarios inspected. What we have, instead, are a number of unsettling situations, and many concerns that need to be carefully balanced. For if there is no clear ethical barrier uniformly outraged by human cloning, so too there seems to me no plausible case that developing and disseminating human reproductive cloning technologies is demanded by any unmistakable moral imperative. There may be a *technological* imperative operating here, but that is quite another thing.

From an ethical point of view, I think, the development of a policy regarding human cloning cannot be settled by the decisive application of clearly determinate principles, but rather requires prudent judgment. Human cloning might console some people in their grief; it might relieve some of the fears of bearing children with serious handicaps; it might contribute to destabilizing heterosexist biases about the family. But it can also offer adults a set of benefits at the cost of risks to the welfare and the dignity of children, and it can more deeply instill in us a penchant for biological ways of marking human significance that may be particularly troublesome in a time when our more serious moral need is to expand our sympathies beyond the biological.

In light of the reasonable concerns that reproductive cloning elicits, and the alternatives available to address the values that it might serve, we'd do better to resist whatever allure it may have. Such a resistance doesn't need to take the form of criminalization; in fact, the problems surveyed here probably don't justify such a coercive measure. Yet even diverse communities have ways of expressing disapproval effectively—in the funding priorities of its public research–sponsoring organizations; in reasoned declarations by centers, committees, and commissions; in the codes of professional ethics promulgated by societies of the relevant practitioners; and in what might be called the general sense of the community, as created by informed public deliberation about the value of biological relationships, of families, and of children more generally. One of the benefits of an approach of this kind is that it allows a certain kind of social flexibility: exceptional cases and new motivations can emerge and make a case for themselves; such instances of reproductive cloning as take place can be observed for their tendency to corroborate either our fears or our hopes. What's more, avoiding a legislative response nudges the debate away from a myopic focus on what people do or do not have a right to do, making central what are prudent and responsible ways to exercise our rights. A better appreciation of this distinction—a growth in our public deliberative powers—would constitute a significant step forward in how contemporary culture decides to use its growing biological powers.

ACKNOWLEDGMENTS

Thomas Murray conveyed an invitation to present my views on cloning and the family to the National Bioethics Advisory Commission, and I expect he did more than simply serve as the messenger. I much appreciate his interest in what I'm trying to do. I also am grateful to Hilde Lindemann Nelson for challenging discussions of cloning—Sara Ruddick and William Ruddick need to be thanked in this connection as well. Carolyn Ells, now assistant professor of bioethics at McGill University, was very helpful as well back in the days when she was my research assistant at the University of Tennessee, before completing her doctorate.

NOTES

1. For discussion, see Steve Minz and Susan Kellogg, *Domestic Revolutions: A Social History of American Family Life* (New York: Free Press, 1989); William J. Goode, *The Family* (Englewood Cliffs, N.J.: Prentice-Hall, 2d ed. 1982); and Stephanie Coontz, *The Way We Never Were* (New York: Basic Books, 1992).

2. For further discussion of the Ayala case, see Hilde Lindemann Nelson

and James Lindemann Nelson, *The Patient in the Family* (New York: Routledge, 1995).

3. Private conversation with William Ruddick, professor of philosophy, New York University (March 1997).

4. For general accounts of sociobiology, see Edward O. Wilson, *Sociobiology: The New Synthesis* (Cambridge, Mass.: Bellnap Press of Harvard University Press, 1975); Peter Singer, *The Expanding Circle: Ethics and Sociobiology* (New York: Farrar, Straus & Giroux, 1981).

5. James Lindemann Nelson, "Genetic Narratives: Biology, Stories and the Definition of Family," *Health Matrix* 2, no. 1 (1992): 71–83.

6. For information on the children of donor insemination, see Jeffrey M. Shaman, "Legal Aspects of Artificial Insemination," *Journal of Family Law* 18 (1980); Patricia P. Mahlstedt and Dorothy A. Greenfield, "Assisted Reproductive Technology with Donor Gametes: The Need for Patient Preparation," *Fertility and Sterility* 52 (1989); Erica Haimes, "Gamete Donation and Anonymity," *Bulletin of Medical Ethics* 6 (1991).

7. See Elise L. E. Robinson, Hilde Lindemann Nelson, and James Lindemann Nelson, "Fluid Families: The Role of Children in Custody Arrangements," in *Feminism and Families*, ed. Hilde Lindemann Nelson (New York: Routledge, 1997).

8. For a general discussion of the ethical significance of vulnerability, see Robert Goodin, *Protecting the Vulnerable* (Chicago: University of Chicago Press, 1985); and, for a critical comment, Margaret Urban Walker, *Moral Understandings* (New York: Routledge, 1998), especially chapter 4, "Charting Responsibilities." For a discussion of the nonvoluntaristic groundings of familial duties, see Hilde Lindemann Nelson and James Lindemann Nelson, "Frail Parents, Robust Duties," *Utah Law Review* 1992, no. 3 (1992): 747–63.

9. I'm here invoking the theme of "moral luck," an idea discussed by moral philosophers interested in circumstances in which persons seem blameworthy for events whose moral character they did not cause (e.g., the responsible truck driver example) or seem excused from blame on the basis of seemingly irrelevant reasons. Contrast public attitudes toward the drunk driver who runs over a child with attitudes toward the equally drunk driver who has the luck to get home without incident. See Bernard Williams, "Moral Luck," in his collection *Moral Luck: Philosophical Papers 1973–1980* (Cambridge: Cambridge University Press, 1981).

10. Yury Verlinsky, Svetlana Rechitsky, Oleg Verlinsky, Christina Masciangelo, Kevin Lederer, and Anver Kuliev, "Preimplanation Diagnosis for Early-Onset Alzheimer Disease Caused by V717L Mutation," *Journal of the American Medical Association* 287, no. 8 (27 February 2002): 1018–21.

11. Dena Tower and Roberta Springer Loewy, "Ethics of Preimplantation Diagnosis for a Woman Destined to Develop Early-Onset Alzheimer Disease," *Journal of the American Medical Association* 287, no. 8 (27 February 2002): 1039.

12. Tower and Loewy, "Ethics of Preimplantation Diagnosis," 1039.

13. Martha Nussbaum's short story, "Little C," in *Clones and Clones: Facts and Fantasies About Human Cloning*, ed. Martha Nussbaum and Cass Sunstein (New York: W. W. Norton, 1998) fleshes out some of these concerns.

14. Salvador Minuchin, *Families and Family Therapy* (Cambridge, Mass.: Harvard University Press, 1974).

15. Joel Feinberg, "The Child's Right to an Open Future," in *Whose Child*, ed. William Aiken and Hugh LaFollette (Totowa, N.J.: Littlefield and Adams, 1980), 124–53. For a critical, insightful discussion of this concern and many others touched on in this article, see Robet Wachbroit, "Genetic Encores: The Ethics of Human Cloning," *Report from the Institute for Philosophy and Public Policy* 17, no. 4 (fall 1997).

16. Still, children conceived primarily for the purpose of providing useful body parts to family members do seem to run the risk of a rather distinctive kind of repudiation. For an account of a child conceived as a bone marrow donor and relinquished for adoption immediately after a successful transplant to its elder sibling, see generally B. D. Colen, "The Price of Life," *Newsday*, 11 March 1990, 5.

Index

151

About the Author

James Lindemann Nelson is professor of philosophy and faculty associate at the Center for Ethics and Humanities in the Life Sciences at Michigan State University. He is the coauthor of *The Patient in the Family* (Routledge, 1995) and *Alzheimer's: Answers to Hard Questions for Families* (Doubleday, 1996), editor of *Rationing Sanity* (Georgetown University Press, forthcoming), and coeditor of *Meaning and Medicine: A Reader in the Philosophy of Health Care* (Routledge, 1999).